BODY BY ANGIE

Is Your
Body
Bankrupt?

Learn to
Invest in
Yourself

*If I can do it,
so can you!*

Angie Lustrick, CN, CPT
Certified Nutritionist and ACSM Certified Personal Trainer

Angie's World
5225 Canyon Crest Dr. #62
Riverside, CA 92507

Phone:
(877) 683-0448
(951) 683-0448
Fax:
(951) 683-4381
E-mail: angiesworld123@aol.com

ISBN 978-0-615-34905-3
1. Nutrition 2. Health

Library of Congress Control Number: 2010902564
Printed and bound in the United States of America

Text design and layout by Elisa Bryant

To Bill, Ann, Eddie, Liz, Kevin, Josh, and Clare-
May this book guide you on your health journey

To Arnie & Estelle-
Within lies the secret to successful aging

HERE'S TO YOUR
HEALTH!

—angie

CONTENTS

Acknowledgments

An abundance of gratitude goes to my clients who have supported me, believed in me 100%, and made this book possible.

To my husband, Bill, who reminds me to dream big and aim for the moon because if I land in the stars, I will still be happy.

To my entire staff at Angie's World: Wilma Young, Deanna Bathauer, Paula Wallace, Jason Fyda, Sila Chiochan, Scott Drexler, Zee Beard, and Tammy Fish. Thanks for your support to all my ideas and dreams. I am so grateful to have such an amazing, hard working staff.

To Wilma Young, my business partner, who has been overwhelmingly supportive of this book, often taking home various pieces of the manuscript to read over the weekend to provide insight and guidance. Your dedication to Angie's World is well noted and I am truly grateful.

To Dee Bathauer, for all your support at Angie's World. You have provided me with insight and ideas on what is truly important for this book.

To Paula Wallace, thanks for watching the pocketbook while I was keeping my eye on the prize. You're the best!

To Starkie Sowers, my first nutrition teacher, who introduced me to the works of Dr. Jeffrey Bland. I am forever grateful to you for writing my letter of recommendation to become a certified nutritionist. Thanks for taking the time out of your busy schedule to review my book.

To John Assaraf, Jennifer Bailey, and my friends in the "Having it All Challenge," thank you for believing in me. You have been the wind beneath my wings. It was because of this group that I found the courage to dust off my old book notes and make this book a reality.

To Angela Diaz and Barbara Frantz, my accountability partners, thank you for keeping me accountable and bringing humor to the process.

To Elisa Bryant who patiently worked with me while I changed and re-changed the cover and graphics for this book. You have a fine eye for detail and it shows in all that you do.

To Ron McCaskill who kept after me to write this book.

To Alice Anderson for making me understand the importance of writing my book.

To Linda Sherman for spending countless hours editing my book. Your time is greatly appreciated.

To my mother who convinced me that I was a good writer and who inspired me at a very early age to be a leader. It has been from watching you that I am who I am today.

To Stephanie Lapinski for giving me the inspiration to write and fueling my fire to succeed in life. Your motivational lunches have meant so much to me. You have kept me on track with my business and have always steered me in the right direction.

To Jeff Katke, Ursula Clausing, Barbara Schiltz and the entire Metagenics staff, you have been my "Verizon network" – you are there whenever I need you. From support for an individual client to PowerPoint presentations, feedback, and printouts for this book – thank you!

To Jeffrey Bland, for inspiring me at a young age to become a nutritionist. It's through your work and your books that I decided to take this career path. It has been deeply fulfilling.

To Maggie, my "dogther," for sitting many a night by me while I worked on my book and providing unconditional love and support.

To Andy Pocock, who had nothing to do with this book but still can claim he beat me in the Mission Inn 5K race. ☺

How To Use This Book

Whether you read this book cover to cover or skim it for quick insights, you will be able to get valuable information that can dramatically change the way you feel physically, mentally and emotionally. If you do invest the time to read cover to cover, you will gain knowledge and implement momentum to your transformation. But if you only have the time to review the Chapter Points and Affirmations at the end of each chapter, you will certainly set yourself on the right path and create a positive force in your life while improving your health. You will also notice there is a testimonial section with the stories of people just like you, their struggles and triumphs as they pursue their journey to health. If you find you are having a tough day, this is a great section to reference. Please keep this book in your library because at certain times of your life, when challenges abound, this book can become a support system and a "boost" when you really need one.

Remember, it is a journey you are undertaking not a destination, and I am here to help steer and guide you. May health and happiness be yours!

If I Can Do It, So Can You!

I would never have dreamed that my flabby thighs would make me ten thousand dollars! After my graduation from college with a degree in biology, I landed my first job as a research and development technician for a major dog and cat food company. Because of my interest in animals as well as in nutrition, this was a dream-come-true job: to work on food that would improve the health of our beloved four-legged family members. And it was a dream job, until my own health started to fail. I drove forty-five minutes to get to work and forty-five minutes to get home. Often the commute home was so bad that it would take sixty to ninety minutes. Knowing I would be stressed out when I arrived home, my loving husband would meet me at the door with a martini for me in his hand.

Due to lack of time I also gave up my exercise routines. When I was in college, I had ridden my bike to school and worked as a waitress at night to help offset my tuition. I wore a pedometer once to work and on an average shift, I walked over six miles! I also frequented the gym on campus at least twice a week.

In addition to throwing my gym habits out the window, I also found myself eating the Krispy Kreme donuts my boss provided for us each morning. He had a serious sweet tooth and took the entire lab out at least twice a week for halo halo (an ice cream drink made with exotic fruits), or a boba (a cream and tea drink with large tapioca balls at the bottom of the glass). In addition to our morning and late afternoon sugar fixes, our company rewarded us with lunch at local restaurants when our performance was good. These lunches were always high in calories and weighed heavily on my waistline. After college and only four short months into my new job, I had managed to add twenty pounds of fat on to my five-foot-two-inch frame!

To make matters worse, two months later I needed to have foot surgery. I had apparently broken a bone in childhood that had never healed correctly. Part of the problem was that I wasn't aware that this bone was ever broken and as I grew up, my foot felt like I had a plantar's wart on the bottom. When I finally couldn't stand the pain, I went to a podiatrist.

The doctor had to re-break the bone and re-set it. He placed a metal pin in my foot to keep the bone in place until it healed. Healing took eight weeks. During that time I wasn't allowed to walk on the foot because it could cause the bone to separate and not rejoin. So I sat on the couch day after day watching TV and eating Little Debbie chocolate and peanut-butter wafers.

When I was ready to get back to work, I had to shed my comfortable sweats and put on my work pants. Uh-oh! My pants didn't fit. I was always a girl who could fit into single-digit pant sizes but now, my bottom was well into the double-digit sizes. I had a problem. A big problem.

When I went back to work, I started suffering from nervousness and anxiety. Often I felt I couldn't speak or form words. I would hide in the lab doing testing and hoping that no one would talk to me.

Instead of going away, these feelings of nervousness and anxiety started to get worse and more frequent. I isolated myself from my coworkers and stopped going to social events on the weekend. I knew something was wrong, so I made an appointment with my doctor.

After extensive blood work I was diagnosed with hypoglycemia (low blood sugar). My doctor sat me down and told me if I didn't change my lifestyle that I would have diabetes within the next five years. My mind started racing. As a child, I remembered that my neighbor's grandmother had diabetes and had gone blind. As her circulation worsened, she had her toes removed, one by one. Eventually both of her legs were amputated at her knees. She eventually died of complications due to diabetes. I couldn't let this happen to me!

I decided to take action. I knew of a personal trainer whom I had met while in college. I called him up and asked if he would help me. He agreed and I made a point to see him three times a week before work.

I started to read fitness magazines to keep myself motivated. I found a picture of a girl with amazing six-pack abs and I decided I wanted to look like her. I hung her picture up in my workstation to remind me to hit the gym on my lunch break on the days I didn't see my trainer.

One day while reading a magazine, I saw an ad to enter a transformation competition. It was a three-month competition in which you were required to take before and after pictures in a bathing suit with a newspaper (to show the date). The winner would receive $10,000 plus a trip to the Arnold Classic Bodybuilding Show in Columbus, Ohio. In addition there was an all-inclusive trip for two to the Bahamas and a two-year supply of supplements. As I read this ad, I could feel my heart racing with excitement. I knew this was exactly what I needed to motivate myself to get back into shape.

I told everyone about this competition that I had entered. Most laughed and told me that I couldn't win. They told me that this competition was fake and that the company did it so that more people would buy their supplements. I was told that even if it were a real competition, they would choose a long-legged blonde with big breasts to win, not a short-haired, vertically challenged girl like me.

Despite their negativity, I knew I could win. I even told my trainer that if I did win, I would give him a $3000 bonus from my prize money. He was in. He trained me to win and pushed me past every comfort zone I had. I even joined Team Diabetes to learn how to run a marathon. This was a big deal since I couldn't run one lap around a track without collapsing from an asthma attack.

I first started doing cardio at the gym. I could do only six minutes at a time before my lungs closed up and my face turned bright red. I kept thinking to myself that since I was having this much trouble in my twenties, I was going to be in a world of hurt in my sixties! I couldn't get the image out of my head of an unpleasantly aged lady with an oxygen tank. Not the image I wanted of myself! Joining Team Diabetes provided guidance and discipline to help me learn how to run and strengthen my cardiovascular system. I had two amazing coaches: Bob and Armando. Without them, such a goal would never been possible. They trained me for three months, the same three months that I was competing to win the transformation competition.

Every day I acted like a winner. I told myself that I had already won. As a winner, I knew that I couldn't eat sweets or drink alcohol. I had to stick to the plan 100%. That's what a winner would do. My mental strength was solid. I could go to parties, walk by desserts, and say no to anything that wasn't on my eating plan. I was determined.

My determination paid off. On the last day for MuscleTech to notify the winners, I received a phone call. I did it! I had won! I remember jumping up and down in my family room with tears in my eyes! I did it! I really did it!

After that day my whole life changed. I had a new perspective on life. I no longer felt the passion to test dog food in a laboratory. I wanted to reach out to others who suffered from health and weight problems. I felt so good and I wanted others to feel that way, too.
I quit my job at the dog and cat food company and took a lesser-paying job at a local nutrition store. Having a local job allowed me to work out every morning before work and not have to waste two hours of my life driving in a car to and from work each day. I also started working for my trainer part-time and went back to school to get my ACSM (American College of Sports Medicine) personal training degree from Loma Linda University.

The nutrition store provided me with classes on nutrition and taught me about vitamins, minerals, and herbs. After completing all three levels of training at the store, the nutritionist pulled me aside and said that I should consider going back to school to get my nutrition degree. He saw that I was passionate about eating right and offered to write a letter of recommendation.

I did, indeed, go back to school, received my certified nutritionist degree, and became a licensed nutritionist. During this time I quit working at the nutrition store and went to work full time as a personal trainer.

After working with my trainer for five years, I branched out on my own and created my business in 2001. I called my company Angie's World (www.angiesworld.com) because after I lost the weight, people, indeed, noticed. They also noticed that I was happier, healthier, and full of life. The comment was always, *Well, in Angie's world you would eat this,* or *In Angie's world you would exercise like that.*

Angie's World appeared to be the perfect name for my business. At Angie's World people would learn how to eat right, exercise correctly, and have a winning attitude. From this business name, an acronym was also born: WAET (pronounced like wait or weight). It was a word my clients would use to re-think their food options. It was the pause or contemplation they had before they indulged in a food. WAET stands for *Would Angie Eat That?*

If I Can Do It, So Can You

A WINNER IS SOMEONE WHO IS COMMITTED.

COMMITMENT MEANS "DOING WHATEVER IT TAKES."

WAET STANDS FOR **WOULD ANGIE EAT THAT?**

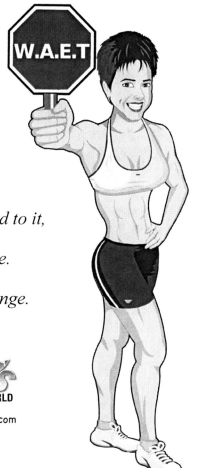

Daily Affirmation

When I put my mind to it,

anything is possible.

I am willing to change.

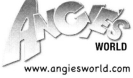

www.angiesworld.com

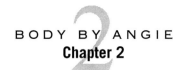

Mindset

Everything happens for a reason. Every single action, whether big or small, makes a difference in this world. From throwing trash out the car window to making a public speech, everything will have an impact.

We are all alive for a specific purpose on this earth. If you believe that you have a purpose, you will realize that certain people, opportunities, and events will come into your life and create situations that shape your thoughts and opinions. These thoughts create new ideas for you and lead you to unique experiences that will ultimately be enjoyable and rewarding. These thoughts will make your life more fulfilling.

You chose this book because you are looking for a change, and it is meant to change your thoughts and opinions about nutrition. Its purpose is to help you gain control of your life by giving you the insight into what it means to eat right so you will eat the appropriate amount of calories from the proper foods. Doing so will give you more energy, more stamina, and better mental clarity so you can achieve whatever it is you are meant to do. Are you ready to begin your journey? Let's begin *now*.

When trying to change your body's dimensions, whether it's releasing fat or building muscle, mindset is crucial for your success. You must believe that you can do it. When you believe it, you can achieve it. It's with this positive mental attitude that you will finally make permanent changes. In my personal story, I had to believe I already was a winner to be able to win.

Imagine yourself at your ideal body weight. Without questioning your thoughts, what was the magic weight you saw in your head? Perhaps this was what you weighed in high school? Your weight before the kids came along? The weight when you were your happiest? Find a picture of yourself at that weight and put it out where you can see it everyday: on your bathroom mirror, on your refrigerator, or by your bed. Having a mental reminder everyday will re-condition your brain to be in synch with your new intentions. Perhaps you have never been at your goal weight. That's okay, too. Look through magazines and cut out pictures of what the ideal you will look like. To make your mental reminder more powerful, make a collage of what activities you will engage in, what foods you eat, and what gives you that feeling you want to achieve when you are at your goal weight.

Say a positive affirmation to yourself each day. Tell yourself, "I weigh ___ pounds and I feel great!" everyday. If you know what body fat percentage you want to be, add that to your affirmation too. Anytime you catch yourself thinking that you are too fat, too skinny, or that you don't like part of your body, I want you to say your positive affirmation. Say it all day long if you need to. You must believe it.

Meditate daily. I first started meditating because I noticed very successful people were doing it. These people were always positive, happy, and motivated. I made the connection that it was their attitude that was influenced by their daily meditations. When I started doing research on meditation, it seemed too good to be true. I had trouble believing that meditation would make me more productive, more focused, more connected to the world and universe, more understanding about others, and the list goes on.

My first thought was, "How can lying or sitting around for thirty minutes to an hour make you more productive?" My type-A personality was telling me that this sounded lazy and counterproductive. But I saw enough people changing positively that I was willing to give it a try.

At first I bought a CD that was thirty minutes long. This fit into my type-A personality nicely because this would give me permission to sit down. I was no longer just sitting; I was listening to a CD. But this was difficult! Right away I realized I had a problem. I couldn't stay awake. My body was conditioned to get out of bed running and continue running with work, house chores, and errands until it was bedtime when my body literally did a crash landing until the next day when the alarm clock greeted me. Relaxation wasn't for me. I couldn't watch TV, a movie, or a concert without falling asleep. When I tried to relax during my day, my mind and body naturally thought it was bedtime.

I picked up on this inability to relax fairly quickly and knew that I needed to address it. Honestly once I identified it, I knew that my current lifestyle was the road to high stress and a possible stroke.

That realization forced me to make a commitment to meditate every day for thirty minutes, whether I could stay awake the whole time or not.

I remember keeping my eyes closed only to peep them open to glance at my watch, "It's only been five minutes...." And again, "Eight minutes, is that it? Thirty minutes is forever!" Somewhere between twelve to fifteen minutes I was asleep.

After two weeks, I finally could stay awake for thirty minutes of meditation. I was able to let go of any thoughts I had of what I should be doing instead —I just let it all go.

And that is when the magic of meditation started to work for me.

All the claims being made about the art of non-doing started becoming evident in my life. My relationships with my clients, friends, and family became strengthened. Perhaps because I was no longer in such a hurry with my daily activities, I was able to enjoy the people around me and appreciate them for who they were. After all, we are human beings, not human doings!

Now that I have been meditating regularly for a year, I know that I will always make time to do it on a daily basis.

I like to think of meditation as inercise; much like exercise, it is needed to strengthen your body. Exercise would be lifting weights and doing cardiovascular activities while inercise would be strengthening your mind and thoughts in a relaxed state.

For those who already exercise, think about how difficult it was to convince your sedentary friends that going to the gym was good for them. It's hard to convey that message because the first couple of times they go to the gym, they are sore, tired, and unable to see the results. It's after being consistent for at least a few months, that the results will be evident.

Inercise is just like that. It takes time to achieve the benefits. It's important to start off slowly, perhaps doing just five to ten minutes per day. Just like the gym, you wouldn't walk in and immediately grab the fifty-pound dumbbells! You would start with the five- or eight-pound weights and over time you would increase the weight size. In fact, you may never grab the fifty-pound weights because your desired look may come with just lifting ten pounds. Just be- cause you meditate doesn't mean you have to become a Zen master to achieve the results you want in your life.

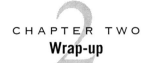

The Mindset

EVERYTHING HAPPENS FOR A REASON.

EVERY SINGLE ACTION, WHETHER BIG OR SMALL,

MAKES A DIFFERENCE IN THIS WORLD.

WHEN YOU CAN BELIEVE IT, YOU CAN ACHIEVE IT.

1. IMAGINE YOURSELF AT YOUR IDEAL BODY WEIGHT

2. SAY A POSITIVE AFFIRMATION TO YOURSELF EACH DAY

3. MEDITATE DAILY

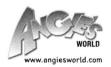

Daily Affirmation

I meditate daily and achieve perfect balance in my life.

I am in the process of positive change.

I am _____ pounds and _____ % of body fat.

ANGIE's WORLD

www.angiesworld.com

Healthy Balanced Eating

How do I know how much I should eat?

This should be the first question that needs to be answered because too much of any food will lead to weight gain. To be able to discuss this, you need to know what a calorie is. A calorie is the amount of heat needed to raise the temperature of one kilogram of water by one degree Celsius at one atmosphere pressure. Unless you are a chemist, this definition means absolutely nothing. So let's come up with a new definition. Our definition should be the amount of energy required to get through our day without gaining weight, yet still provide enough nutrients to make us feel great. So how is this determined? The traditional method would be to weigh yourself, then to use a chart based on height and gender and figure out what your ideal weight should be. This method is poor. It does not take into consideration how much muscle is on your body, whether you have big bones, whether you are an athlete or sedentary, or what your fitness goals are.

This book is designed with simple guidelines to help you achieve optimum health. It is not necessary to purchase any measuring equipment to be able to use this book. However, if you are the analytical type that likes to see numbers, I would like to take the time up front to show you how some simple tools can be used to help you on your fat-releasing journey. In order to get started, my type-A friend, you will need to buy yourself a bioelectrical impedance body weight scale and a set of calipers. (Or you can get your body fat tested by a certified trainer or nutritionist to figure out your percentage of body fat and lean muscle mass.) I recommend both the scale AND the calipers because you will learn two different things:

1. The scale will tell you your body fat percentage (Accuracy depends on the scale you buy but don't worry, most scales are extremely accurate within themselves, meaning if the scale says you were 38% and are now 36%, you know for sure you released 2% body fat).

2. The calipers will tell you about your eating habits and glycogen levels (more on this later). These numbers can be converted by using a chart to tell you what your body fat percentage *is trying* to be based on your eating habits.

So by using the scale, you can determine what your current body fat is, and by using the calipers you can determine what your body is trying to do: burn fat or store fat.

For example if the scale says that you are 38% but the calipers say that you are 45%, then this means that your body is in fat-storing mode, is becoming heavier every day, and will reach a plateau when you are actually 45%.

On the other hand if the scale says you are 38% but the calipers determine that you are 28%, you are in fat-burning mode and will continue to lose weight until your body is at 28% body fat.

A very easy way to determine if you are in either fat-burning mode or fat-storing mode is to see if the calipers are measuring below or above 30 mm.

< 30 mm = fat burning mode
> 30 mm = fat storing mode
20 -30 mm = ideal glycogen levels
< 20 mm = a depleted state, often desired by models and bodybuilders during competition

*Note: The calipers do not measure in body fat percentage; they measure in millimeters (mm). They are measuring your glycogen stores. Glycogen is stored glucose your body uses for its immediate needs. When you eat food or caloric beverages, your body first breaks these calories down into glycogen.

To understand glycogen better, imagine looking at a human skeleton. Now imagine adding muscle on top of that skeletal frame. Now picture yourself pouring honey over the entire muscle system. This thin, yellow, viscous fluid is the immediate energy store for your muscles. Your body only stores glycogen in your muscles and in your liver, with a maximum total of 1000 calories. Once your glycogen stores are maxed out, your body is then forced to store extra energy as fat. In this case, you will see your mm readings above thirty. Your primary focus will be to eat more regularly and not feel stuffed after eating.

If your readings are below 30 mm, this means that you are getting adequate calories in your day and are burning off the calories you are consuming. If this is your situation, your primary focus will be to choose more balanced meals.

If your caliper reading is below 20 mm, you are now in starvation mode. This means that your body requires more food than you are giving it. It is impossible to feel energetic and/or build muscle when your glycogen stores (caliper readings) are this low. Your body is in a catabolic state and is relying on your muscle mass to stay alive. If you fall in this category, your primary focus will be to add more calorie-dense foods to your meals and you may have to eat at times when you aren't hungry.

To calculate your body fat using calipers, you will have to do a conversion. See the table in the back of the book titled "Caliper Body Fat Interpretation Chart" or the chart provided when you purchased your calipers. In this area you can also calculate how many calories you should be eating to release weight knowing your body fat percentage and total calories is not critical for fat loss. Simply following the plan will insure that you are releasing fat and not muscle.

When using your calipers, measure three areas of your body:

A) Your tricep (arm) area
    (back of your arm, using a vertical pinch fold)

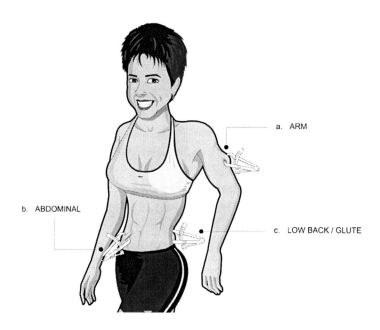

a. ARM

b. ABDOMINAL

c. LOW BACK / GLUTE

B) Your abdominal area (midway between hip and belly button, using a diagonal pinch fold)
C) Your glute area (top of buttocks, near lower back/hip, using a horizontal pinch fold)

Always measure the same side of your body (all right-side, or all left-side measurements). It is easier if you have someone else test you. Make sure you don't over-squeeze the calipers. When you hear the click, stop pinching. The best way to do this is to pull the skin away from the body and then use the calipers.

These three measurements will tell you a lot about your eating habits—as if you didn't already know!
   A) Arm region – this is where you store starches like bread, pasta, rice, and potatoes
   B) Abdominal region – this is where you store simple sugars like alcohol, sweets, and fruits
   C) Low back/glute region – this is where you store fats like fried foods, mayonnaise, cheeses, and nuts

Note: The above case will not be true if you have had liposuction. The body will store fats differently and cannot be accurately determined using this method. If this concerns you, just make sure to get all your numbers below 30 mm by eating a balanced diet.

So if you measured your body and found that you measured above 30 mm in your:
-Arm, then you are eating too much from the starch group
-Pelvic region, then you are eating too many simple sugars
-Glute region, then you are eating too much fat

Conversely if you find that a number is really low in a certain area, you may not be eating enough of those foods. Remember, a healthy caliper reading is between 20 – 30mm.

Now that you know what foods to limit or avoid, we can plan an eating strategy to specifically minimize those problematic areas.

The strategies to releasing fat are simple and easy, provided you follow them. Think of these strategies as investments to your health.

Investment Strategy Number 1: Eat every two to three hours.

Investment Strategy Number 2: Eat a protein with every meal.

Investment Strategy Number 3: Never go to bed hungry.

Investment Strategy Number 4: Drink enough water.

Investment Strategy Number 5: Move!

These are the five golden rules. These strategies will move your body from overweight/unhealthy to healthy weight/healthy body. In this chapter we will cover the first three strategies.

If your intention is to become a fitness fanatic and have an athletic looking body, a few more investment strategies will apply:
Bonus strategy #1: Avoid added sugars & alcohol.
Bonus strategy #2: Weight train three times a week.

STRATEGY #1: Eat Every Two to Three Hours

Start by getting a clean sheet of paper and writing at the top left corner of the page the time that you normally wake up. Underneath that time, write down the time it would be thirty minutes after waking. This should be your breakfast time. Then write down the time three hours after each time for the rest of your day. Give yourself about four lines of space between each of the times you write.

SAMPLE DAILY EATING PLAN

6:00 am – wake up

6:30 am – breakfast

9:30 am – snack

12:30 pm – lunch

3:30 pm – snack

6:30 pm – dinner

9:30 pm – snack

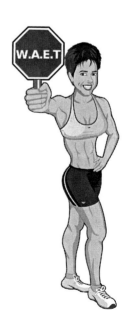

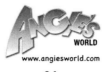

www.angiesworld.com

It is very important that you eat within thirty minutes of rising. The word breakfast means *breaking the fast*. The fast is the eight hours you sleep without eating. The sooner you eat breakfast, the sooner you will turn your body into a fat-burning machine. You will realize that the sooner you eat, the sooner you will get hungry again in your day. That's because your metabolism is working for you, burning away fat and that takes calories (more food)! The opposite is also true: If you skip breakfast, you won't feel hungry until much later in the afternoon. That's because your body is still in fasting mode and is holding onto the calories you ate the night before.

A common mistake is to skip breakfast or skip multiple meals when trying to release weight.

This is a HUGE mistake! The heaviest people I see are those who only eat one time a day, the second heaviest eat twice a day, and the average body type eats only three times a day. The leanest people I see eat five to six meals per day. They eat small portions and never allow themselves to get weighed down by huge meals. Think about children: Their natural instinct is to snack all day long, eating a few things here and there and they are naturally energetic and lean. It isn't until we teach them to eat only three meals that their bodies change and start storing fat. How does that work? When we eat, we speed up our metabolism. Think about a bonfire at the beach. The fire is much like your metabolism. Let's say we decide to have a party at the beach and I put you in charge of keeping the fire going. If you wanted that fire to burn all night, you would have to throw a few logs on the fire every few hours. If not, the fire would go out. So, as the party goes on, you become distracted and forget about the fire. Oops! Now you are in trouble; the fire is down to embers, and you don't want me to find out. So you quickly throw a huge bundle of logs on top of the fire in the hope that the fire will return back to its normal level. This is much like forgetting to eat after four hours, and now your body is starving, so you eat an over abundance of food.

So what happens? At the beach you will smother your fire, the embers do not have the energy to burn all that wood and now you have white smoke. In your day this would represent a high-fat, high-calorie meal that you gobbled down really fast, leaving you feeling tired, lethargic, and ready for a nap. But it gets worse. You stopped your metabolism and now your body is at a standstill and will not burn body fat until things get back to normal. Just like the fire on the beach after you smothered it, the fire will start to rekindle and a few hours later… *whoosh*! The fire has ignited in full force. The flames are higher than before and finally will go back to normal if the fire is fueled properly. This is much like what happens in your body. You will feel a rush of insulin from eating a large amount of food and then will return to normal. If you were to live your life this way, the constant fluctuation between high sugar levels (high insulin) and low sugar levels (low insulin, the crash after the highs), will keep your body in a constant state of distress. Your body wants balance and will start holding onto fat during your eating frenzies because it is not sure when the next meal will come. The body starts storing *everything* for those famine times! Yikes! So when we eat regularly every two to three hours, our blood sugar levels remain balanced, our bodies no longer feel the need to store calories, and we can now release the fat from our bodies. Remember, we want to release the fat, not lose fat. Human nature, like the body, will always try to find what it's lost, but when we release, we let it go for good.

Now that we understand strategy #1, let's go over strategy #2.

STRATEGY #2: Eat A Protein with Every Meal

Now that we know we have to eat every two to three hours, we have to decide which foods we will be eating during those times. Protein is important because it breaks down into amino acids, which are the building blocks to our health. Amino acids make up hair, skin, nails, the lining of our digestive tract, and muscles. Without amino acids, our bodies cannot repair themselves.

Protein can come from animal or vegetable sources. Here's a list of protein choices I recommend:

CONCENTRATED PROTEIN

Serving size: 3-4 oz. cooked, or as indicated

(1 serving = approximately 150 calories)

Meat, poultry, and fish should be grilled, baked, or roasted; fish may also be poached

Keep cheese intake low due to saturated fat

- Eggs, 2 whole, or 3 egg whites plus 1 whole egg

- Egg substitute, 2/3 cup

- Fish, shellfish, 3 oz. fresh or 3/4 cup canned in water

- Poultry: chicken or Cornish hen (breast only), turkey

- Leg of lamb, lean roast

- Beef, very lean (5% or less fat); buffalo, venison, elk

- Tofu, 5-6 oz. or 1 cup (fresh), or 2-3 oz. cube (baked)

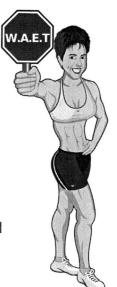

- Tempeh, 3 oz. or 1/2 cup - Seitan, 1/3 cup

- Soy or veggie burger, 4 oz.

- Cottage cheese, nonfat or lowfat, 3/4 cup

- Ricotta, part skim or nonfat, 1/2 cup

- Mozzarella, part skim or nonfat, 2 oz. or 1/2 cup shredded

- Parmesan cheese (grated), 6 tbsp.

Plan your meals around the protein of your choice. How much protein should you have? Take a look at your hand. The palm of your hand is your minimum protein requirement per meal. The size of your full hand (palm + fingers) is your maximum amount of protein needed per meal. The thickness of the meat should be equivalent to the thickness of your hands. For a thicker cut, fold your fingers over your palm to determine the size that is appropriate for you. Athletes should eat the full hand serving while sedentary or less active individuals need only the palm size amount of protein.

For those of you that have a difficult time with protein, you can opt for a protein shake or bar to meet your needs.

Once you have established how much protein is right for you, add carbohydrates and fats to that meal. Note that the strategy is about protein. It is okay to eat protein alone as a snack, but never just carbohydrates or fat by themselves. The exception to this is if you are eating within two hours of a protein meal. For example, when I get up in the morning I do not have much of an appetite so I start my day with a protein shake with water. Once my body starts waking up, an hour later I eat oatmeal with fruit and nuts. Then two hours after that I eat one egg with three egg whites and beans. My carbohydrates (oatmeal and fruit) where consumed between two meals that were high in protein and less than two hours apart. When you incorporate carbohydrates into your diet, you do not have to measure with a scale or measuring cup. The easiest way is to take your hands and make two fists. One fist is for a starch (bread, pasta, rice, potato, or bean) and the other fist is for a non-starch (all vegetables). Starchy food items have more calories so you must obey the fist rule for these items. This means that the *maximum* amount of starch you should eat at one serving is the size of your fist; you may eat less. On the other hand, the other non-starchy foods are so low in calories that your *minimum* requirement is one fist; you may eat more. The calories in these foods are so low that by the time you have digested them, you have burned more calories than are actually in the food! Here is a quick guide to starchy versus non-starchy veggies. Category 1 vegetables are non-starchy vegetables. Try to eat at least 2 cups of them per day!

Category 2 vegetables, grains, and legumes are starchy vegetables. Try to limit these food groups to one fist or smaller per meal.

If you are interested, please visit stopchronicdisease.com to find a nutritionist or naturopathic doctor that can determine the exact number of starchy vegetables that are right for you.

CATEGORY 1 VEGETABLES

FREE FOOD! The calorie count in these foods is so low that by the time you digest them, you have burned more calories than you consumed!

Serving size: 1/2 cup - min. 3-4 servings unlimited

Fresh juices made from these are allowed (1 serving = approximately 10-25 calories)

- Artichokes • Asparagus • Bamboo shoots
- Bean sprouts • Bell or other peppers
- Broccoli • Broccoflower • Brussels sprouts
- Cabbage (all types) • Cauliflower • Celery
- Chives • Cucumber
- Eggplant • Garlic • Green Beans
- Greens:
    bok choy, escarole, Swiss chard, kale, collards, spinach, dandelion, mustard and beet greens
- Leeks
- Lettuce/Mixed greens:
    romaine, red and green leaf, endive, spinach, arugula, radicchio, watercress, chicory
- Mushrooms • Okra • Onion • Radishes
- Salsa (sugar-free) • Scallions • Sea vegetables (kelp, etc.)
- Snow peas • Sprouts
- Squash: zucchini, yellow, summer, spaghetti
- Tomatoes or mixed vegetable juice (low sodium)
- Water chestnuts, 5 whole

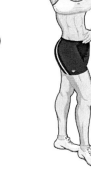

CATEGORY 2 VEGETABLES

Serving size: 1/2 cup, or as indicated (1 serving = approximately 45 calories)

- Beets, winter squash (acorn, butternut)
- Carrots, 1/2 cup cooked or 2 medium raw or 12 baby carrots
- Sweet potatoes or yams, 1/2 medium baked
- Yukon Gold, new or red potato, 1/2 medium

GRAINS

Serving size: 1/2 cup cooked, or as indicated

(1 serving = approximately 75-100 calories)

- Basmati or other brown rice, wild rice
- Barley, buckwheat, groats, or millet
- Bulgur (cracked wheat)
- Quinoa
- Teff
- Whole oats, raw, 1/3 cup; cooked oatmeal 3/4 cup
- Whole wheat, spelt, or kamut berries
- 100% whole wheat, spelt, or kamut
- Whole grain rye crackers, 2 each
- Bread: mixed whole grain or 100% whole rye, 1 slice
- Whole wheat tortilla or pita, 1/2
- Low-carb tortillas, 2 small or 1 large
- Kashi® 7 Whole Grain Puffs cereal, 1 cup

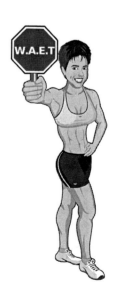

THE MAGICAL FRUIT: BEANS

Despite the lyrics, beans are an important part of your diet. They are high in protein and in fiber. Dietary fiber helps balance blood sugar levels and lower cholesterol levels naturally. Fiber also causes satiety, making you feel full after a meal. Other good sources of fiber are bran, brown rice, nuts, and green vegetables. If you are having a difficult time incorporating fiber into your diet, you may need to take a powdered fiber supplement.

Beans should be eaten every day, one to three servings, depending on your caloric needs, a serving being ½ cup.

LEGUMES

Serving size: 1/2 cup cooked, or as indicated (1 serving = approximately 110 calories)

• Beans:

> garbanzo, pinto, kidney, black, lima, cannellini, navy, mung,
>
> fat-free refried, green soy beans

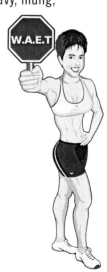

• Bean soups, 3/4 cup

• Hummus, 1/4 cup

• Split peas, sweet green peas, lentils

You will notice that I did not include corn on the lists. Corn is very high in sugar and creates fat to store around the belly (visceral fat). I do not recommend corn in your eating plan. Corn became a staple in the American diet during the depression; before that, it was meant to fatten the cattle and pigs. Mothers began feeding their children corn to fatten them up so that they didn't become too thin and die. Corn is sweet so it was well tolerated by kids. You might find reference in numerous books that a family was so poor that their children were corn-fed. In books about that era, you'll find children from very poor families referred to as "corn-fed" so after the Great Depression, many of our traditional family recipes contained corn. Interestingly enough, Europeans never added corn to their diets. Recently I had a client visit Europe for her summer vacation. While she was driving with her family one day, she saw rows and rows of corn and thought how wonderful it would be to eat their corn. At night they stopped at a restaurant and were surprised that corn was not on the menu even though they were surrounded by corn fields. She told the waiter, "I don't see corn on the menu. It's obviously in season, why can't I find it?" The waiter quickly replied, "Madam, the corn is for the pigs!"

Carbohydrates are necessary in a balanced eating plan. They contain vitamins, minerals, anti-oxidants, phytonutrients, and other compounds that we are just now beginning to discover in research laboratories. Carbs help your body stay alkaline, which means on a pH scale our bodies favor a more basic balance, opposed to being acidic. Acidity is very hard on our bodies. An acidic state promotes cancer and disease in the body.

When the Atkins' diet was popular, you may recall everyone was *trying* to go into ketosis, a very acidic state! Ketosis occurs when carbohydrates are not present in the body. Depending on a person's glycogen stores (stored carbohydrate energy), this can take anywhere from three to seven days. When these carbs are depleted, the body goes into ketosis, where the liver converts fats into fatty acids, which can be used for the body for energy. It is not a naturally occurring state for the body; it is a defense mechanism to stay alive when carbohydrates are scarce. The ketone bodies that are released during this reaction are released in the urine and the breath (it smells much like alcohol). Some medical resources regard ketosis as a physiological state associated with chronic starvation, and it is often regarded as a crisis reaction of the body. It is potentially life-threatening and causes destruction of muscle tissues.

Think about the word carbohydrate. When you break it down, you will notice the word *hydrate.* Carbohydrates help our body hold onto water so that our cells do not dry out. Often when people are on a low-carb diet they will lose weight very fast but they are not just losing fat, but also water and muscle. You will notice that once a person begins to eat carbs again, they will practically blow up over night. This is caused by the body's inability to process carbs. The pancreas will need to start producing amylase again. Amylase is an enzyme needed to breakdown carbohydrates. During the time when the pancreas is remembering how to produce amylase, our bodies will undergo an inflammation response. To make matters worse the body will try to maintain balance and not go back to that ketosis state by holding more hydration than before the body underwent the low-carb diet. This results in a hyper-saturated state that can take up to three months to return to balance.

Using the starch guide above, let's look at what a lunch including a sandwich might include. Open up one of those fists and you will realize that for most of us, the size of our hand is equivalent to just one slice of bread. Add a palm or full hand serving of protein to that ½ sandwich, and don't forget the other fist. It will fill you up with the non-starchy foods like lettuce, tomato, pickles, sprouts, and cucumbers. Finally, add a thumb size amount of fat into your diet. Choose good fats and avoid the bad fats.

A detailed list of good fats:

OILS AND NUTS

GOOD FATS

Serving size: 1 tsp, or as indicated
Oils should be cold pressed
(1 serving = approximately 40 calories)

Plant Oils

Avocado (fruit), 1/8
Coconut milk, light, 3 tbsp.
Coconut milk, regular, 1 1/2 tbsp.
Flaxseed oil (refrigerate)
Olives, 8-10 medium
Olive oil, extra virgin (preferable)
Cooking Oils
Olive oil
Canola oil
Coconut oil, 1 tsp
Ghee (clarified butter) 1 tsp.
Grapeseed oil, 1 tsp.
Earth Balance® spread, 1 1/2 tsp.

Nuts & Seeds:

Serving size as indicated
(1 serving = approximately 100 calories)
Almonds or hazelnuts, 10-12 whole nuts
Coconut, unsweetened grated, 3 tbsp.
Peanuts, 18 nuts or 2 tbsp.
Pine nuts, 2 tbsp.
Pistachios, sunflower, pumpkin, or
   sesame seeds, 2 tbsp.
Walnut or pecan halves, 7-8
Nut butter, 1 tbsp. made from above nuts

BAD FATS

Deep Fried Foods
Hydrogenated Oils
Lard
Yellow Cheeses
Margarine
Mayonnaise

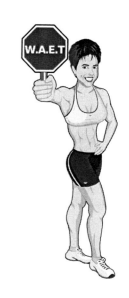

FirstLine Therapy®

Good fats contain vitamins (A, E, and K) and/or essential fats (Omega 3, 6, and 9), which are needed in your body for brain production (memory and focus), eye health, skin hydration (from the inside out), blood sugar regulation, blood clotting, and pain reduction. But most importantly, they help rid the body of bad fat.

You might recall in the 80's when everyone was on a low-fat diet kick. You might have noticed this worked great for those who were already skinny, but it did nothing for those trying to lose body fat. The reason is that you need good fat to get rid of bad fat (like attracts like). To give you a visual, think of your heart connecting to your veins and arteries. Now think of those veins and arteries like they are big water slides transporting blood to every square surface of your body. When you eat bad fat, it tends to stick to the walls of your waterslides. Much like gum on a sidewalk, if not removed the gum will harden and will never come off. In the body, we call this atherosclerosis, or hardening of the arteries. Now think of the good fats, like rafts that are floating down the waterslides. Because they are attracted to bad fats, they will scoop up these bad fats before they harden and put them on their back (on top of the raft). The raft eventually makes its way to the liver where the bad fats are processed, broken down, and removed from the body via elimination.

I also like to think of the good fats as nature's lubricant. If your joints are cracking and aching or if your eyes and hair are dry, you need to lube them up. Increase the essential fats in your diet and you will be amazed how quickly your joints, eyes, and hair recover. Now, look at your elbows. Are they dry and scaly? This is another indicator that you are low in oil. I think of my elbows as my oil sticks. When the oil stick is dry in your car, your car needs oil. Much the same as your car oil stick, your elbows will always tell you if you need oil. If the skin on your elbows is soft and naturally moisturized, then your oil is at a healthy level.

For insurance, I take fish oil capsules twice a day. Make sure the fish oil capsules you buy contain a purity symbol on the label. Otherwise you may also be buying heavy metals that will toxify your body (lead, cadmium and mercury).

Fruit should also be in your eating plan. Typically a person wanting to release weight should eat no more than two servings of fruit per day. An athlete or person wanting to add muscle to his or her frame may need three to four servings of fruit a day. Overeating fruit will have the same effect as eating too much sugar, but more on this later! But not to fret: A fruit serving is a fairly generous portion.

FRUITS

Serving size as indicated (1 serving = approximately 80 calories)

- Apple, 1 medium
- Apricots, 3 medium
- Berries:

    blackberries and blueberries, 1 cup; raspberries and strawberries, 1 1/2 cups
- Cantaloupe, 1/2 medium
- Cherries, 15
- Fresh figs, 2
- Grapefruit, 1 whole
- Grapes, 15
- Honeydew melon, 1/4 small
- Mango, 1/2 medium
- Nectarines, 2 small
- Orange, 1 large
- Peaches, 2 small
- Pear, 1 medium
- Plums, 2 small
- Persimmon, 1/2
- Tangerines, 2 small
- Watermelon, 2 cups

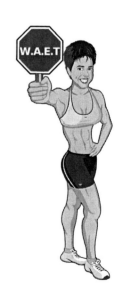

FirstLine Therapy

If you wanted to eat only two servings of fruit per day, you could have three apricots and two small nectarines to make up your two servings.

*Note that bananas and pineapple are not on the above list. These fruits are extremely high in sugar and will have a tendency to store around your waistline as fat.

I also do not recommend eating these fruits unless they grow in your environment. This means that you will either need to buy your local fruits when they are in season and can them for the winter, or do as I do, and eat foods only when they are in season. When you eat fresh fruits and vegetables that are locally grown, you are helping your immune system. Let me explain. When a plant grows in your environment, it is exposed to the same stressors your body is being exposed to like pollution, smog, electromagnetic chemicals, and/or water tainted with lead, arsenic, cysts, and pharmaceutical drug by-products. The plant will produce phytonutrients that will protect the plant from being harmed from these outer influences. Thus, when you eat these plants, your body is receiving the nutrients specifically to help protect you from any harmful substances in your environment.

The final food category is dairy and dairy alternatives. Dairy should be minimized in your diet, with most females needing just one serving per day while most males will require two servings per day. Dairy is high in sugar and is hard to digest. You may be thinking that you will not get enough calcium in your diet by minimizing this category. While dairy products are a great source of calcium, they are not the only source. In fact, some other calcium-rich foods include sesame seeds, hazelnuts, sardines, salmon, dark leafy green vegetables, broccoli, butternut squash, sweet potato, raisins, dried figs, and enriched soy or rice milk, to name a few. Here is a list of serving suggestions for dairy and dairy alternatives:

DAIRY/DAIRY ALTERNATIVES

Serving size: 6 oz., or as indicated (1serving = approximately 80 calories)

- Almond milk, plain, 8 oz.

- Buttermilk, nonfat, 1% or 2%

- Hemp milk, plain, 6 oz.

- Milk, nonfat or 1%, 6 oz., Soy milk, plain, 8 oz.

- Sour cream, nonfat, 6 tbsp.

- Yogurt (soy), plain unsweetened, 4 oz.

- Yogurt (also goat milk or Greek), plain unsweetened, 6 oz. nonfat

- Fat-free feta cheese, 2 oz.

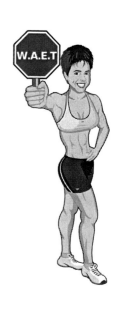

FirstLine Therapy®

Finally when making food choices, make sure that you choose a variety of colors. Each color provides different nutrients for your body. Most of us are creatures of habit and will eat the same fruit every day. Break that habit. Not only will you benefit from different nutrients but think about this: Different pesticides are used on different fruits and vegetables (unless you are eating organic!); therefore, if you eat the same fruits and vegetables, you are receiving the same pesticides in your body each day. The FDA has stated that pesticides are safe in low doses. Your body has a better chance of removing pesticides in lower concentrations from your body.

Here is a quick glance of what the color of fruits and vegetables mean:

RED- Improves circulation and cleans blood, maintains a healthy heart, reduces risk of prostate cancer, reduces tumor growth, lowers LDL cholesterol, supports joint tissue, urinary tract health, memory function, and has powerful antioxidants

BLUE/PURPLE- brain food: increases memory function and focus, reduces inflammation, lowers risk of stroke and heart disease, promotes healthy aging, and supports urinary tract health

YELLOW/ORANGE- Improves eye sight, reduces risk for macular degeneration, promotes collagen formation, maintains healthy mucous membranes, and maintains a healthy immune system

GREEN- lowers cancer risks, normalizes digestion, boosts immune system, increases vision health, reduces risk of cataracts, and maintains strong bones & teeth

WHITE- helps white blood cells, lowers blood pressure, promotes healthy cholesterol levels and heart health

(No, M&Ms don't count! ☺)

STRATEGY #3: Never Go to Bed Hungry

This is a very controversial strategy. Most nutritionists will tell you not to eat anything after 6 or 7 P.M. But what if you stay up until 2 A.M.? This would break our first strategy to eat every two to three hours. Regardless of what time you go to bed, you should never go to bed hungry or feel hungry at any time, for that matter.

Nutritionists will suggest that you don't eat past a certain time because most people are conscious of what they put in their mouths during the day, making health-minded choices for breakfast, lunch, and dinner when they are trying to release weight. But when they sit in front of the television, they begin to mindlessly snack. Bags of chips or cookies can get polished off without them realizing how much was consumed. But if you are mindful about what goes into your mouth, evening snacking is not a problem. I prefer a protein snack before bed. Carbohydrates can cause blood sugar levels to elevate and are known to cause nightmares, so avoid starchy carbohydrates within two hours of bedtime. Fruits and vegetables are okay before bed but remember the protein rule!

My favorite nighttime snacks are a glass of soymilk, a protein shake (you can add fruit to make a smoothie), or scrambled egg whites with salsa.

Another reason you do not want to go to bed with your stomach growling is because when you're hungry, your body shuts down its growth hormone production due to lack of nutrients. Growth hormone is responsible for building muscle and burning fat while you sleep.

When we go to bed with protein in our stomach, we tend to sleep more soundly and are more likely to achieve the 7 to 8½ hours of sleep our bodies need. However, if you go to bed hungry, chances are you will wake up from a growling stomach or be restless due to your body being under stress from starvation mode.

Wrap-up

Healthy Balanced Eating

TOO MUCH OF ANY FOOD WILL LEAD TO WEIGHT GAIN.
THE INVESTMENT STRATEGIES TO RELEASING FAT ARE...

STRATEGY NUMBER 1: EAT EVERY TWO TO THREE HOURS.
STRATEGY NUMBER 2: EAT A PROTEIN WITH EVERY MEAL.
STRATEGY NUMBER 3: NEVER GO TO BED HUNGRY.
STRATEGY NUMBER 4: DRINK ENOUGH WATER.
STRATEGY NUMBER 5: MOVE!

BONUS STRATEGY #1: AVOID ADDED SUGARS & ALCOHOL.
BONUS STRATEGY #2: WEIGHT TRAIN 3 TIMES A WEEK.

EAT PROTEIN WITH EVERY MEAL:
   PALM SIZE IF SEDENTARY, FULL SIZE HAND IF YOU ARE ACTIVE.
EAT ONLY LOCALLY GROWN FRUITS AND VEGETABLES, IF POSSIBLE
   — PREFERABLY ORGANIC.
EAT ALL THE COLORS OF THE RAINBOW-
   EACH COLOR HAS A DIFFERENT EFFECT ON THE BODY.

GOOD FATS AND CARBOHYDRATES ARE NECESSARY TO ACHIEVE
   OPTIMUM HEALTH.
NEVER GO TO BED HUNGRY BUT DON'T EAT CARBS BEFORE BED
   EITHER. (PROTEIN IS YOUR BEST CHOICE).

Daily Affirmation

I choose healthy and balanced foods.
I nourish my body with quality nutrition.
I release fat and gain lean muscle every time I eat.

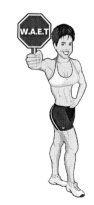

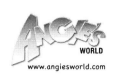

WORLD
www.angiesworld.com

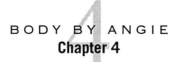

Important Nutrients & Other Factors

When your body starts to respond to your new eating plan, it is normal for you to get anxious and want to continue seeing results at a faster and faster rate. To insure that your results do not plateau, you will want to address these other factors: water, foundational supplementation, and hormone balance.

STRATEGY #4: Drink Enough Water

Since our bodies are made up of about 70% percent water, our body's water requirements need to be replenished throughout the day to keep working properly. Our bodies naturally lose water through sweat, evaporation, and urination. When someone becomes dehydrated, it means the amount of water in his or her body has dropped below the level needed for normal body function. Next to air, water is the element most necessary for survival. We can go without food for almost two months, but without water, we can only stay alive for a few days. Dehydration can be caused by losing too much fluid, not drinking enough water or fluids, eating too many salty or processed foods, and excessive alcohol consumption. Our bodies also lose fluid from sweating, vomiting, diarrhea, and fever. Diabetics often have excessive urine output which puts them at greater risk of dehydrating.

Special considerations need to be made for children and the elderly. Children are more susceptible to dehydration because of their smaller body weights which cause a faster water and electrolyte turnover. The elderly often become dehydrated due to thinner skin, which makes it harder for their body to retain fluid due to poor thermoregulation (temperature regulation). Also the elderly often don't like to drink fluids because of incontinence issues.

Common symptoms of dehydration are low urine output or very dark urine, dry or sticky mouth, dry or sunken eyes, muscle cramps, a drop in body temperature after exercise, confusion, dizziness, and lethargy. Rapid heart beat and feeling faint when standing up quickly may be caused by lack of fluids. You may use a simple test to check this: pinch your skin and if it springs back into position immediately, you are well-hydrated.

Did you know that 75% of Americans are chronically dehydrated? It has been estimated that half the world population is dehydrated. Why is this so? Is it because there is a lack of fluids available? The answer is no. The reason is that the thirst mechanism is so weak that it is often mistaken for hunger. So it is very common for people to overeat because they are thirsty. In fact one glass of water will shut down midnight hunger pangs for almost 100% of dieters.

But overeating isn't the only problem caused by a lack of water; even mild dehydration will slow down one's metabolism as much as three percent. So, even if you aren't overeating due to thirst, you may gain weight. Also a mere drop in body water by two percent is the main cause of daytime fatigue and can cause fuzzy short-term memory, trouble with basic math, and difficulty focusing on the computer screen or on a printed page.

Without water we'd be poisoned to death by our own waste products because when the kidneys remove uric acid and urea, these must be dissolved in water. We even need water to breathe. Our lungs must be moist to take in oxygen and excrete carbon dioxide. Most people have no idea how much water they should drink. The average human requirement is eight to ten, eight-ounce glasses of water per day. An inactive person in a cool climate may need less, while an athlete training in the desert will need much more. Overweight people should drink an extra glass for every twenty-five pounds they exceed their ideal weight. (An easy way to determine your water consumption needs is to take your total body weight and divide by two. The number is the amount of water in ounces you need to drink.)

It is better to get your fluids in small sips throughout the day instead of drinking large amounts at once. Electrolyte solutions are the best for quenching thirst and replenishing your cells. Sports drinks are not advised because of the amount of sugar they contain. Coaches should educate their team players on the importance of drinking electrolyte fluids that are low in sugar. Fluids should be encouraged before, during, and after a game or practice. If you believe that dehydration is developing, consult a doctor before the person becomes moderately or severely dehydrated. Coaches should also be aware that many sports enhancement supplements such as creatine, caffeine, and protein powders can put an extra burden on kidneys and put a team player more at risk for dehydrating.

Some athletes, such as wrestlers or bodybuilders who need to reach a certain weight to compete, dehydrate themselves on purpose to drop weight quickly before a big game or event by sweating in saunas or using laxatives or diuretics, which makes them go to the bathroom more. This practice usually hurts more than it helps. Athletes who do this will feel weaker which affects performance. They can also have more serious problems, like abnormalities in the salt and potassium levels in the body. Such changes can also lead to heart rhythm problems or kidney failure.

Dieting can also sap a person's water reserves. Beware of diets or supplements, including laxatives and diuretics, that emphasize shedding water-weight as a quick way to lose weight. Losing water weight is not the same thing as losing actual fat.

Research has shown that drinking enough water throughout the day can significantly ease back and joint pain for up to eighty percent of sufferers, decrease the risk of colon cancer by forty-five percent, slash the risk of breast cancer by seventy-nine percent, and lessen the risk of developing bladder cancer by fifty percent.

While dehydration is a serious risk during warm weather, it is possible to drink too much water. A condition called hyponatremia can occur when excess fluids are consumed. This condition is caused by excess loss of electrolytes (sodium, potassium, calcium, magnesium, and phosphates), through urine. Though not as common a problem as dehydration, hyponatremia is a considerable threat. An electrolyte imbalance can be fatal.

Considering the benefits of drinking water, it is important to keep in mind my favorite adage: Everything in moderation. Just because something is good for you doesn't mean that a whole lot more will be better. Listen to your body.

Drinking water is smart and can help your body perform at its peak, whether it is mental clarity or athletic performance you are seeking.

If you purchased a bioelectrical scale for your house, you probably know by now that your new bathroom scale tells you your body water percentage. These scales will slightly under report your actual hydration levels. A fully hydrated female's, hydration level will be between fifty to fifty-five percent, and a fully hydrated male will be between fifty-five to sixty percent. If you are checking your hydration levels and are consuming more water, you should notice that these levels will slowly reach their desired percentage within three months. However, if you are not noticing any increase in your hydration status week after week despite your increased fluid intake, you may have another underlying issue. Often the cause is either a deficiency of electrolytes in your body or a protein deficiency.

Electrolytes are the minerals your body needs to absorb fluids. These minerals are calcium, magnesium, phosphorus, potassium, and sodium. They are responsible for activating the electrical tissue of your body, which are both your muscle tissue and your neurons. Muscle contraction is dependent on electrolytes and, if deficient, your muscles will experience weakness and severe muscle contractions. Commonly this is reported as severe cramps in your toes or legs.

If your eating plan is low in protein, your body will be deficient in amino acids. If your muscles are deficient in amino acids, they will lose their ability to absorb water. My clients who are experiencing this tell me that they are drinking water all day long, yet they can't seem to get enough, and they are urinating all day long. The fluids they are drinking are not being absorbed and are flowing right through their bodies, which can create a bigger electrolyte imbalance.

If you are experiencing any of these symptoms, you may want to increase your electrolyte and protein intake. If you are concerned, contact a certified nutritionist to help you balance these issues.

In addition to electrolytes and protein, it is important to take foundational supplements. Foundational supplements are the supplements your body needs to achieve optimal health. These supplements are a multivitamin, a fish oil supplement, and a probiotic. If you are over thirty years of age, you may also consider taking CoQ10.

A multivitamin is necessary if you can answer yes to *any* of these questions:

1. Are you under stress?
2. Do you frequently skip eating vegetables in your diet?
3. Do you not eat your two servings of fruit each day?
4. Do you eat fast food on a regular basis?
5. Are you skipping meals?
6. Are you sick or do you frequently get sick?
7. Do you suffer from a chronic disease or illness?
8. Do you consume alcohol or caffeine?
9. Do you smoke?
10. Are you taking any prescription or over-the-counter medications?
11. Are you injured or have you recently had surgery?
12. Are you pregnant or breast feeding?

If you answered yes to any of these, you will need to take a multivitamin once a day.

If you answered yes to more than three of these, you will need to take a multivitamin twice a day. And if you answered yes to five or more, you should be taking a multivitamin three times a day.

When choosing a multivitamin, chose one from a reliable company. Don't buy the cheapest ones you can buy; this is your health we are talking about! If you want cheap, you can find online websites that have supplements for as little as one dollar. I don't know about you, but this freaks me out. God save us all if we are choosing poor-quality, low-budget vitamins to put into our systems! Think about this: The bottle and the lid that the vitamin comes in cost money; the label they put on the bottle costs money; the cotton they put inside the bottle as well as the safety seal cost money. So what's inside the bottle? How much could they possibly spend on the actual vitamin?

Read the label! If you notice food colorings or dyes in the product, do not take them. There is no reason to have pretty-looking vitamins when all you are going to do is swallow them. Food colorings and dyes contain chemicals that can cause brain disturbances. If you notice that the product has a lot of the minerals bound to oxides or carbonates, this is another clue that your vitamin is of poor quality. Carbonates are very cheap to buy and are poorly absorbed in the body. Carbonates translate to more profit for the vitamin company. Calcium carbonate is a prime example. This type of calcium is known to cause bone spurs and blocks absorption of many nutrients in the large intestine! If you notice that your vitamin has sugar in it, throw it away! Manufacturers will add this to make you feel more energetic! You will see sugar listed in *Other Ingredients* under the secret code names of sucrose, corn syrup, high fructose corn syrup, and maltodextrin.

The key to understanding your vitamins is to start reading the label, not the fancy hype on the front of the bottle. This was a hard lesson for my client, Debbie.

Debbie had been seeing me for nutrition counseling on a monthly basis. She was following the eating plan and was losing body fat, but she still wasn't feeling well. I noticed that every time she came in, my BIA machine showed that her toxic load was increasing. This didn't make much sense to me since her eating was so clean. I went over the list of possible suspects: Excess caffeine? No. Artificial sweeteners? No. Pain medication? No. Antibiotics? No. Hmmm. New prescription? No. I was stumped. She then showed me the vitamins she had been taking, purchased from a vitamin shop. She thought they should be good because there was a doctor's name on it. I asked her if she knew the doctor and she said no. I then asked to look at the ingredient list. BINGO! We found the toxic ingredients she had been consuming! Inside her multivitamin were food colorings (red #40, blue #2, yellow #5), sugar in three different forms, many carbonate forms of vitamins including calcium carbonate, and the icing on the cake— *talc!*

Yes, you read that correctly: *talc*, the stuff you put on babies' butts. I couldn't understand why talc would be in a multivitamin so I looked it up in one of my favorite books, "Food Additives" by Ruth Winter, M.S. This is what Ruth says about talc:

TALC: Fresh chalk. Magnesium Silicate. The lumps are known as soapstone of steatite. An anti-caking agent added to vitamin supplements to render a free flow and also to chewing-gum base. Gives a slippery sensation to powders and creams. Talc is finely powdered native magnesium silicate, a mineral. The main ingredient of baby and bath powders, face powders, eye shadows, liquid powders, protective creams, dry rouges, face masks, foundation cake make-ups, skin fresheners, foot powders, and face creams. It usually has small amounts of other powders such as boric acid or zinc oxide added as a coloring agent. Prolonged inhalation can cause lung problems because it is similar in chemical composition to asbestos, a known lung irritant and cancer-causing agent. There is no known acute toxicity, but there is a question about it being a cancer-causing agent upon ingestion. It is suspected that the high incidence of stomach cancer among the Japanese is due to the fact that the Japanese prefer that their rice be treated with talc. Talc is not considered food grade by the FDA as it contains asbestiform minerals.[1]

Wow! Maybe you should take a look at your vitamins! At Angie's World, we carry the purest products that are GMP-certified (Good Manufacturing Practice) and NSF-certified (National Standard Federation). These certifications mean that third-parties go into the supplement companies manufacturing plants to make sure that the place is clean (free of bugs, debris, for example) and that each pill you take gives you exactly the dose it claims on the bottle. Without third-party testing you are relying on the vitamin company to tell you the truth. How honest do you think some of these companies are? How much actual nutrition do you think you are getting for that dollar?

Fish oil is another foundational supplement. Fish oil contains Omega 3 fatty acids (such as EPA and DHA), that are essential for the body. Essential means that your body cannot make these fatty acids; it must get them from your diet. Some of the benefits of consuming fish oil (or flax, if you are vegetarian) include:

- healthy skin, hair, nails, and eyes
- balanced blood sugar levels
- anti-inflammatory properties and pain management
- improved cardiovascular health
- releasing body fat
- cognitive function, memory, and focus

Remember to choose a fish oil supplement that is purity-certified to be free of heavy metals, pesticides, and other contaminants.

The ratio of EPA to DHA is important. If you are trying to reduce inflammation in your body or assist your body in releasing weight, you will want to have six times more EPA than DHA in your supplement. If you are trying to improve eye health or memory,

49

you will want to have a 1:1 ratio of EPA to DHA. If you are interested in all the benefits without emphasis on a particular benefit, you will want to find a 3:2 ratio of EPA to DHA. Please reference the *Tracking Your Progress* section and look for the EPA & DHA supplement chart for more information.

You also should take a probiotic every day. The term probiotic refers to friendly bacteria that are normally found in your intestines. The good bacteria is responsible for:

- detoxifying the intestines
- strengthening the immune system
- improved digestion function
- regular bowel movements
- aiding your body's ability to absorb and/or synthesize essential fatty acids and vitamins
- producing natural antimicrobials that prevent the growth of harmful bacteria and fungi
- preventing the formation of carcinogenic compounds in the colon
- creating beneficial acids, which promote a healthy intestinal pH
- helping in maintaining healthy cholesterol levels

Unfortunately our unhealthy lifestyles of excessive alcohol intake, stress, and exposure to toxic substances like smog, paint fumes, poor quality food (fast food) and other chemicals can drastically decrease the amount of these active cultures living in our gut. Even normal aging can disrupt the balance of friendly bacteria and can lead to poor health.

In addition, antibiotics will wipe out the healthy flora inside your gut. While antibiotics are necessary in certain situations to fight infections and unhealthy bacteria, repeated use can contribute to increased susceptibility to infection and intestinal dysfunction. And the bad news is that bad bacteria grow three times faster than healthy bacteria. That means, if you are currently on or have recently used antibiotics, your gut is highly susceptible to being re-infected. The best way to stop re-infection is to take a probiotic during antibiotic use and to continue for at least one month after finishing your antibiotics. And whatever you do, do not stop your antibiotics early after deciding to take them! You must finish the full dose to completely eradicate the infection you are fighting. If you don't, two things can happen: You won't kill the bad bacteria completely and you are very likely to be re-infected. If this happens, you will need a stronger antibiotic to kill off the bad bacteria a second time. Or you will kill off the infection enough where your own immune system wipes it out *but* not fast enough and you become an unhealthy bacterial donor to all your friends, family, and co-workers. The bad news is that this bacteria may become resistant to antibiotics which makes it harder for newly exposed people to fight it off.

Other factors that diminish healthy bacteria in your gut are:

- If you are taking antacids or other gastric acid inhibitors (when you take medications that reduce stomach acid, you are allowing unhealthy bacteria to grow where they would otherwise would not)
- If you eat a high fat or low fiber diet (a poor diet makes it difficult for health promoting bacteria to thrive)
- If you travel abroad (foreign travel increases your risk of exposure to intestinal parasites and bacteria that upset the natural bacterial balance)
- If you are exposed to food and water contaminants (chlorine [think Splenda], pesticides, antibiotics, and others). We often unknowingly consume compounds that alter the intestinal environment

You may think that all you have to do is eat yogurt. Though it is beneficial to include yogurt in your diet, yogurt contains only *some* active cultures, the main culture being acidophilus. But there are many cultures: each with its own benefit. Some are used for Irritable Bowel Syndrome, others for bloating or inflammation, others for pain or discomfort in the lower abdominals. I would also like to mention that a quality probiotic supplement will contain between five and sixty billions active cultures, depending on the culture. When you eat yogurt, a typical serving will provide one billion active cultures. Thus, you may need to eat up to sixty servings of yogurt to achieve the desired result! New research, however, shows that active cultures cannot live in pasteurized milk. Meaning, the manufacturer may add these friendly bacteria to the yogurt but by the time you consume this yogurt, all or many of the cultures will be dead.

All good bacteria will boost the immune system but each active culture (probiotics) performs different tasks inside the gut:

- Lactobacillus acidophilus: helps maintain normal balance of the intestines, irritable bowel syndrome, bloating, diarrhea, cramping, flatulence, bad breath, combats vaginal yeast and Candida overgrowth
- Lactobacillus salivarius: prevents and fight H. Pylori, helps breakdown undigested protein
- Lactobacillus paracasei: calms digestive upsets, assists other probiotic strains, improves absorption of nutrients and lipids
- Lactobacillus plantarum: helps irritable bowel syndrome and pain associated to IBS, helps preserve omega 3 fatty acids and other nutrients, helps eliminate potentially pathogenic microorganisms
- Bifidobacterium lactis: blocks toxic effects of wheat gliadin, improves absorption of nutrients, and assists in breakdown of dairy products
- Bifidobacterium bifidum: improves symptoms of diarrhea and constipation, aids in synthesis of B-vitamins and absorption of calcium
- Bifidobacterium longum: keeps digestive system running smoothly, blocks the growth of harmful bacteria, ferments sugar
- Streptococcus thermophilus: alleviates symptoms of lactose intolerance and other GI disturbances

There are also beneficial prebiotics. Prebiotics are foods that are introduced into your system that feed and stimulate the growth of the good bacteria in your body. Prebiotics are the nutrients needed to keep your good bacteria alive in your intestines. Active cultures feed off prebiotics and are more likely to establish a culture in your intestines if food is provided for them. The most common prebiotics are fructooligosaccharides (FOS) and inulins. They are naturally occurring polysaccharides (indigestible sugars) found in asparagus, barley, chicory root, garlic, honey, Jerusalem Artichoke, jicama, leeks, onions, tomatoes, and wheat. FOS is also used as an alternative sweetener, having a sweetness level between 30 – 50% of sugar.

Several studies have found that FOS and inulin promote calcium absorption in both the animal and human gut. The intestinal microflora in the lower gut can ferment FOS, which results in a reduced pH. Calcium is more soluble in acid, and, therefore, more of it comes out of food and is available to move from the gut into the bloodstream.

Another important consideration to achieving your ideal body is to make sure your hormones are balanced. My company provides Biomeridian testing that can determine what hormones your body needs to balance. I like to think of hormone balancing like making your favorite recipe. It takes multiple ingredients in different amounts to come out with a masterpiece. Altering the ingredients even slightly will alter the masterpiece. The approach that the pharmaceutical companies take is that we all should eat the same size TV dinner. Take a look around you; we are not all the same size. Often the portion is too big and the ingredients are too processed. A better approach to hormone balancing would be to give your body all the specific ingredients necessary to make your perfect masterpiece! When a client comes in and we determine a hormone imbalance, I will provide ingredients such as DHEA, black cohosh, evening primrose, phytoestrogens, phytosterols (phyto means plant-based), and soybean concentrate. Each person's supplementation and dosage would be different based on his or her needs. Then as the body becomes more in balance, it is important to re evaluate their "recipe" and remove or replace the ingredients to continue the balance.

Keep in mind that hormone changes are normal as we age. And yes, men have hormones too! The medical field likes to treat menopause and low testosterone production as a disease. It is not. Menopause, for example, is a normal transition in a woman's life. Often the pharmaceutical hormones will prolong menopause, so a woman will be in menopause for five to ten years! A healthy menopause lasts two to four years.

Another factor associated with fat release for women is xenoestrogens. Xenoestrogens are end product metabolites of estrogen in the body. Estrogen is naturally stored in the fat cells of our bodies. When a woman starts to lose weight, an increase of estrogen is released into her bloodstream. As the estrogen is utilized the xenoestrogen starts accumulating in her system. These xenoestrogens are responsible for mood swings and emotional disturbances. Often what is necessary is a natural supplement that removes these xenoestrogens safely from the body. One such supplement that you could add to your daily regimen is indole-3-carbinol, which is found in cruciferous vegetables, a.k.a. broccoli, cauliflower, brussels sprouts, and cabbage. So it would make sense to add these to your eating plan and/or the supplement daily, especially during menopause.

Once you have addressed your hormone imbalances, it is important to eat right, drink plenty of water, manage your stress levels *and* exercise to keep the body in balance.

Nutrients and Other Factors

TO DETERMINE YOUR BODY'S DAILY WATER INTAKE:
TAKE YOUR TOTAL BODY WEIGHT (IN POUNDS) AND DIVIDE BY TWO.
THIS IS THE NUMBER OF OUNCES YOUR BODY NEEDS DAILY.

REMEMBER, WE WANT TO RELEASE THE FAT,
NOT LOSE FAT. HUMAN NATURE
HAS IT THAT WHEN WE LOSE SOMETHING,
WE ALWAYS TRY TO FIND IT!
WHEN WE RELEASE, WE LET IT GO FOR GOOD.

CHOOSE A MULTIVITAMIN WITHOUT ARTIFICIAL COLORS,
SUGARS, AND WITH LITTLE OR NO OXIDE
AND CARBONATE FORMS OF VITAMINS.

FOR OPTIMUM HEALTH; A MULTIVITAMIN,
FISH OIL SUPPLEMENT, AND
PROBIOTIC ARE ESSENTIAL.

CHOOSE A PROBIOTIC BASED ON WHAT HEALTH
PROBLEM YOU ARE EXPERIENCING.

Daily Affirmation

Drinking water helps me to feel happier and healthier.

I gain energy by my choices of food and supplements.

I select only quality products to build my body and nourish my brain.

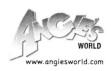

WORLD
www.angiesworld.com

Beware of Sugar and Alcohol

Sugars and alcohol can be major pitfalls when trying to transform your body or release weight. They both have the potential to be extremely addictive, sabotage hours of hard work in the gym, and cause major health problems.

When I am leaning out for a photo shoot or figure competition, I take sugar and alcohol completely out of my diet. This even includes fruit, fruit juices, and wine. Leaning out is a term bodybuilders and fitness models use to describe the process of removing excess glycogen and water from their bodies so that muscle definition and tone is apparent. This weight is not fat weight since the athlete or model is already lean. Usually the weight lost is about five to ten pounds from their normal weight.

When I am not taking pictures, I will allow myself to eat two servings of fruit a day and an occasional drink, usually on the weekends. A larger person can certainly tolerate three fruits per day.

Sugar is a very high glycemic food, which means it spikes your blood sugar (glucose) very fast. This high level of blood sugar causes your pancreas to release large amounts of insulin to digest the sugar. The sugar is then absorbed into the cell and causes a major drop in blood sugar levels. This drop creates the feeling of hunger and cravings for more high-glycemic foods so that your blood sugar becomes normalized. When the blood sugar level spikes again, this process is repeated. This vicious cycle will repeat over and over and over, often until your body becomes insulin insensitive which is eventually diagnosed as diabetes. High blood sugar levels can cause hyperactivity, anxiety, difficulty concentrating and crankiness. Low blood sugar leads to mood swings, fatigue, and headaches.

Maintaining a proper balance between blood sugar (glucose) and insulin levels is essential for optimum health. Too much glucose will eventually lead to disease but too little will cause low energy levels and confused thinking (Your brain needs glucose, too!). Balanced glucose and insulin levels support:

- energy levels
- weight and body fat content
- healthy HDL cholesterol levels
- healthy triglyceride levels
- healthy blood pressure
- overall cardiovascular health
- delicate tissues, such as the eyes
- nervous system health, especially peripheral nerves
- healthy growth hormone levels

The trouble with eating sugar is that once you eat it, your body craves more of it. Have you ever noticed that when you get back from a vacation where you allowed yourself to have sweets, all you want is more sugar? It takes two weeks of avoiding sugar to get rid of the cravings. This means that if you allow yourself a bite here and a bite there, you will always crave sugar. Those who avoid sugar often report little or no cravings for sugary things and feel energized and emotionally balanced.

Sugar increases not only your risk of diabetes but also obesity, disease, and certain cancers. Sugar increases your risk for Crohn's disease and ulcerative colitis. It has even been linked to causing asthma, arthritis, heart disease, appendicitis, multiple sclerosis, hemorrhoids, varicose veins, osteoporosis, emphysema, atherosclerosis, gout, Alzheimer's disease, epileptic seizures, and metabolic syndrome.

Sugar suppresses your immune system. Bacteria and yeast feed on sugar. Therefore you are more likely to stay sick longer when stricken by these foreign invaders. Is that cookie really worth it?

According to the USDA data, people who consume high levels of sugar in their diet have the lowest intakes of essential nutrients, especially vitamin A, vitamin C, folate, vitamin B-12, calcium, phosphorus, magnesium, and iron. Vitamin A is important for keeping your skin, eyes, mucus membranes, and lungs moist. Vitamin C's benefits range from boosting your immune system to fighting the common cold and warding off deadly disease, like cancer. It's a potent antioxidant, helps with collagen production, fights off gum disease, and speeds the healing of wounds. Folate's primary function is to aid the brain and neural function. It also helps regulate homocysteine levels in the body (High homocysteine levels may have an effect on atherosclerosis by damaging the inner lining of arteries and promoting blood clots. It may lead to stroke in people with existing heart disease). Vitamin B-12 helps with energy levels, emotional stability, mental clarity, and healthy homocysteine levels.

Sugar upsets the mineral relationships in the body, which results in chromium and copper deficiency, along with interfering with calcium and magnesium absorption. It can even lower the amount of Vitamin E in the blood. Interestingly enough, chromium is found in animal foods, seafood, and plant foods, but not in refined starches (sugars). Your body needs chromium to regulate blood sugar. Copper is a mineral found in small amounts in all body tissues. It is responsible for deactivating free radicals in the body, which are unstable by-products of a cell causing damage to the body tissues. Copper also helps your body absorb iron, speeds the healing of wounds, assists in collagen formation for healthy, firm skin, helps maintain a normal heartbeat, and boosts the immune system. Copper is provided in a healthy eating plan containing nuts, seeds, organ meats, shellfish, and whole grains. Calcium and magnesium are minerals found in larger amounts in our bodies. They are partially responsible for building strong bones thereby reducing your risk of osteoporosis, aiding in muscle relaxation and contraction, electrical stability and nerve conduction, and maintaining vascular tone. Vitamin E has tremendous anti-oxidant capabilities, also helping to

remove free radicals from your body. It is also a cholesterol reducer, immune booster, skin protector, and inflammation reducer in
the body. Vitamin E works with magnesium and calcium to regulate
hormones. So instead of taking each individual mineral listed as a
supplement, you would be better off ditching the sugar habit, taking one multi-vitamin per day, and maintaining a balanced nutrition
plan.

Sugar accelerates the aging process. When sugar is consumed,
it attaches itself to proteins in a process called glycation. Once a red
blood cell is glycated, it can not convert back to a healthy cell. You
must wait until your body produces new blood cells; this process
takes up to ninety days. Glycated molecules contribute to the loss
of elasticity found in aging body tissues. The more sugar in your
blood, the faster the damage takes hold. Sugar can also make tendons more brittle.

Sugar causes tooth decay and gum disease. When sugar sits on
your teeth, it creates decay faster than any other food substance. It
can contribute to saliva acidity and lead to periodontal disease. Once
swallowed, sugar creates an acidic digestive tract. Sugar can even
cause constipation. It is also responsible for causing food allergies
and lowering the ability for enzymes to function, causing indiges-
tion. It has even been linked to gastric cancer.

Sugar can cause poor protein absorption; it can change the structure of protein and impair the structure of DNA—our genetic make-
up. It is so powerful that it can permanently alter the way proteins
act in the body. In fact, certain tests are used to help doctors understand how your body is being affected by dietary sugar. A fasting five-hour glucose tolerance test can be performed as well as the
glycated hemoglobin test (HbA1c). The glucose tolerance test is
performed on an empty stomach. You are then given 75 –100g of a
sugary drink to consume. Your blood is then tested every hour, for
five hours. In a normally functioning body, this test causes stress on
the body but no side effects. In a weakened body, this test will cause
shakes, sweating, dizziness, fainting, and could lead to death, but

the test is always stopped before that happens! This was the test that was used to determine my pre-diabetic state when I was diagnosed with hypoglycemia. It was very uncomfortable for me and I almost passed out. I was so sick after the test that I had to eat real food before I left the lab. It took me almost another hour to recover. I had to call in sick that day because I just couldn't function. That test really opened my eyes to how sick I had become from eating high amounts of sugar in my diet. I fast-forwarded in my mind what my future would be. I saw myself sick and tired. I was already feeling ill, what would it be like at forty, fifty, or sixty years of age? The other test, The HbA1c test is performed every three months because that is how long it takes for your body to produce new red blood cells (RBCs). The HbA1C test is not as difficult or as long and is performed with a simple blood test. It will test your hemoglobin, which is the oxygen-carrying pigment that gives blood its red color. About 90% of hemoglobin is hemoglobin A. When we eat sugar, the sugar binds to our RBCs and glycates them, which means they permanently change their structure and ability to perform normal tasks. An impaired glucose tolerance level is anything greater than 5.6. The closer you get to 6, the more diabetic. Your body has to create new normal blood cells taking up to ninety days to give your body fresh, clean blood (provided you don't continually eat sugar during this time, which would repeat the process). Note that HbA1C is not affected by short-term fluctuations in blood glucose concentrations, for example, due to meals. It is affected by continuous sugar in your diet. It's not that you can never have sugar again. You just don't want to consistently bombard yourself with it. This is one of the reasons that, when starting a personal training program, a trainer tells you it will take three months before you see a noticeable difference in your body. Your RBCs must be healthy and performing optimally to be able to physically change your body.

Sugar can damage many organs of the body, including the liver, the pancreas, the kidneys, and the adrenal glands. The liver can be damaged in several ways. It can increase the size of the liver by making the liver cells divide, it can increase the amount of liver fat and it can cause liver tumors. The pancreas can have problems due to excessive insulin secretion used to break down the sugar in your body. It has even been linked to pancreatic cancer in women. Your kidneys may increase in size and produce pathological changes. It may even lead to the formation of kidney stones and can adversely affect urinary electrolyte composition. It has been linked to renal cell carcinoma, which is cancer of the kidneys. And your adrenal glands lose their ability to function with sugar. Adrenal glands sustain your natural energy throughout the day. If you wear them out with excess sugar, you no longer have your natural get up and go. This results in a vicious cycle.

Do you have a problem balancing blood sugar? Take the quiz!
1. Do you feel tired and sluggish after you eat?
2. Do you carry excess weight around your abdomen?
3. Are you concerned about your blood pressure?
4. Are you concerned about your triglyceride levels?
5. Do you frequently lack energy?

If you answered yes to any of these questions, this may be related to your blood sugar balance.

Regular exercise helps maintain blood sugar and healthy insulin sensitivity, as well as healthy body fat levels. Excess body fat appears to play a strong role in insulin activity.

Nutrients that support healthy blood sugar are: CLA (conjugated linoleic acid), Omega-3 essential fatty acids, alpha-lipoic acid, magnesium, chromium and cinnamon.

You might think after reading this that it is better to eat artificial sweeteners instead of sugar. Absolutely not! Your body knows how to break down sugar. It has been around since the beginning of man and the body recognizes it and does a great job removing it from your system. Artificial sweeteners, on the other hand, are very new and are looked upon as foreign chemicals in your body. When artificial sweeteners enter your body, your body treats them as a toxin. But it is actually worse than that. Artificial sweeteners do such a good job making our bodies think that we are eating sugar that our pancreas will start secreting insulin as soon as the chemical hits our tongue. In the absence of sugar, insulin will make you store body fat! Then to really make matters worse, when you decide to eat real sugar, your brain no longer calculates it as having calories. Now your body won't send any signals to stop eating sugar and sweets. This puts your body into total metabolic confusion! Artificial sweeteners are not broken down like a normal sugar molecule; instead they are taken to the liver to be broken down like a toxin. The liver has to break down all toxins in the body and, if it becomes overloaded, these toxins may escape back into your bloodstream and imbed themselves in other tissues. Toxins are acidic to your body and an acidic environment promotes cancer and disease. When toxins start to accumulate inside your tissues, your body tries to protect itself by pulling the toxins out and storing them in your fat cells (Oh, and by the way, your brain is mostly made up of fat, too! This means toxins can be stored there also). We normally think of fat cells as stored energy sites, but they actually have a second role: storing toxins. When the toxic load becomes too high for a fat cell two things can happen: a) you will produce more fat cells to store toxins or b) your body will have to transfer water from muscle cells to help neutralize the acid inside the fat cells by surrounding them with water. You may understand this more if you can visualize a water balloon and how it feels when you hold it from the bottom. Now touch an area where fat concentration is high on your body (under the arms, inner thigh, behind the knee, or under your chin and neck). If it feels like the water balloon, then your issue may be toxic burden, not fat overload. For people experiencing toxic overload it becomes almost impossible for you to release weight because your body would much rather hold onto the fat-containing toxins than to release the fat and re-introduce the toxins back into the system. Please read the chapter on detoxification for further clarification on this subject.

Some of the most common artificial sweeteners are aspartame, saccharin, acesulfame potassium (k), and sucralose.

Aspartame, also known as NutraSweet or Equal, and acesulfame potassium (k) are two hundred times the sweetness of sugar. Saccharin, also known as Sweet n' Low, is three hundred times sweeter. Sucralose, also known as Splenda, is six hundred times sweeter than sugar. The term excitotoxins is used to describe these mega-sweet chemicals. These are substances (usually amino acids) that react with specialized receptors in the brain in such a way that they lead to destruction of certain types of brain cells. MSG (monosodium glutamate) and hydrolyzed vegetable protein are also known excitotoxins. Another problem with consuming excitotoxins is that your taste buds adapt to the hyper-sensations. Then when you eat regular sugar or a piece of fruit, it tastes extraordinarily bland and tasteless. It can take weeks for your body to lose its hypersensitive palate.

Aspartame was re-approved by the FDA on October 22, 1981 after first being approved in 1974 and then pulled from the market. It was pulled for further testing to determine if it might cause brain damage and tumors. It is used in breath mints, chewing gum, hard candy, instant coffee and tea beverages, non-alcoholic beverages, fruit juice-based beverages, concentrates, syrups, glazes, and icings.

Acesulfame K was approved by the FDA on July 27, 1988, despite the warning by the Center for Science in the Public Interest (a Washington D.C.based consumer group) stating that the animals in the studies suffered more tumors than the control group. Acesulfame K is found in chewing gum, dry beverage mixes, confections, canned fruit, gelatins, puddings, custards, and in some diet drinks.

Saccharin has been in use since 1879. It is used in mouthwashes, dentifrices, and lipsticks. On March 9, 1977, the FDA banned its use in foods and beverages because it was found to cause malignant bladder tumors in laboratory animals. There was an immediate outcry led by the Calorie Control Council (an organization made up of commercial producers and users of saccharin). Then the FDA, urged by Congress, delayed the ban. The moratorium on prohibiting the use of saccharin has been extended indefinitely. Since 1977, however, saccharin containers carry labels warning that saccharin

may be hazardous to your health. Saccharin has exhibited muta-
genic activity (genetic changes) and the FDA has concluded that
it is carcinogenic to animals and is potentially carcinogenic to humans. In 1997 the Calorie Control Council successfully requested
the National Toxicology Program to review new data to which led to
a delisting of saccharin as a carcinogen.

Sucralose, also known as Splenda, is an artificial sweetener made
from sugar. It has no aftertaste and is more stable. The FDA approved its use in April 1998. It is used as a tabletop sweetener,
in baked goods, fruit spreads, desserts, confections, and diet beverages. Splenda is made by removing three hydrogen-oxygen groups
from the sugar molecule and replacing them with three molecules of
chlorine. You wouldn't go outside and drink down your pool, would
you?

Many products contain artificial sweeteners and a healthy body
can deal with small amounts of them. It's the consistent daily bom-
bardment of these chemicals that can place an extra burden on your
body and makes it harder to release weight.

When looking at sugar content on a food label, try to find a product with 12 grams of sugar or less per serving. This sugar must
come from natural sugars, not ADDED sugars. No added sugar is
acceptable for the body. Natural sugar comes directly from fruit, like
raisins or dates. This is the safe amount that your body can digest at
one sitting.

I personally try to avoid all artificial sweeteners. Instead I will
opt for stevia, agave nectar, honey, molasses, or brown rice syrup
first, and all in moderation!

Stevia is an herb that is characteristic of its sweet leaves. It's a
member of the mint family originating in Paraguay. Its sweetness is
two hundred times sweeter than sugar and has been shown to benefit
tooth health. It has been known and used in South America for over
four hundred years without ill effect and has been used for more
than thirty years in Japan. The United States has known about stevia
since 1918, but industry pressure from the sugar trade has blocked

its use. This herb is quite adaptive and is capable of being cultivated in diverse climates, not just in South America. It now is FDA-approved but as a food supplement, not as a food additive. New food supplements such as Truvia are now emerging on the market. Truvia is made from erythritol, rebiana, and natural flavors. Erythritol sounds like a chemical but it's actually a naturally fermented sugar alcohol found in grapes and pears. It's made by a culture in a process like making yogurt from milk. Rebiana comes for the sweetest part of the stevia plant.

Agave nectar, or agave syrup, is a sweetener commercially produced in Mexico from several species of agave, including the same plant that makes tequila! It is sweeter than honey but less viscous. It consists primarily of fructose and glucose. It is low glycemic and can be used by diabetics.

Honey is 100% pure and a natural sweetener made and stored in honeycombs by the honey bees. Nearly one million tons of honey is produced worldwide each year. It is believed that honey has been consumed and farmed by humans as far back as ten to twenty million years ago and the practice of beekeeping to produce honey dates back to at least 700 BC. Honey has many health benefits ranging from antiseptic, antioxidant, and cleansing properties. It is also used to heal cuts and wounds, and in skin care and beauty products.

Molasses is a viscous byproduct of the processing of sugar cane or sugar beets into sugar, cane molasses and sugar beet molasses, respectively. Blackstrap molasses is just one type of molasses made by processing refined sugar cane into table sugar. It is rich in many minerals, including iron, calcium, potassium, magnesium, copper and manganese.

Brown rice syrup, also known as rice syrup, is a sweetener derived by culturing cooked rice with enzymes (usually from dried barley sprouts) to break down the starches, then straining off the liquid and cooking it until the desired consistency is reached. It is a relatively neutral flavored sweetener that is roughly half as sweet as sugar or honey.

Interestingly enough, sugar can lead to alcoholism. Research shows that many alcoholics are actually addicted to the sugar in alcoholic beverages, not the alcohol itself! Alcohol can pack on the pounds fast because it is high in calories and is delivered in a liquid state that can be ingested quickly. Alcohol contains seven calories per gram. This may mean nothing to you, but consider this: Protein and carbohydrates contain only four calories per gram. Alcohol has almost twice the calories as those foods. The only higher caloric substance would be fat, weighing in at nine calories per gram.

One of the problems alcohol has is that it lowers your inhibitions when you drink it. Often people will be conscious of their eating but once a few drinks are consumed, they start over-eating the trail mix or mixed nuts provided at the bar. Or the appetizers start to look really tempting despite the fact that they are usually deep-fried and laden with cheese.

Another problem with alcohol is that it disrupts sleep when consumed in high doses. Initially it will relax a person into falling asleep but will awaken you later in the night due to the sugars in the alcohol.

Although there is a debate among experts over whether alcoholism should be considered a disease, the National Institute on Alcohol Abuse and Alcoholism recognizes it as such. Chronic alcohol abuse increases a person's risk for developing serious health problems, such as liver disease, high blood pressure, heart disease, stroke, cancer (especially cancer of the esophagus, mouth, and throat), and pancreatitis. Liver disease is characterized by inflammation and scarring (cirrhosis) which is irreversible. The liver is the only organ that doesn't notify us of its problems until it is too late. Because alcohol is extremely toxic to the body, your liver stops breaking down fat and other toxins, and starts to work immediately on the alcohol. During this time, the liver is not able to adequately maintain blood sugar levels. It takes up to seventy-two hours for alcohol to be completely removed from your system, meaning you are no longer burning body fat! So consider this: If you drink every Friday, Saturday, and Sunday, it will take up to Wednesday to remove the alcohol completely out of your system. This leaves you with just Thursday to release body fat. And remember, you can only release half a pound of fat per day! What a waste of six days!

When consuming large amounts of alcohol, it impedes the digestion of food because it decreases the secretion of digestive enzymes from the pancreas. It also inhibits the absorption of nutrients in the blood. Over time this can lead to malnutrition.

The U.S. Department of Health and Human Services and the U.S. Department of Agriculture recommend that alcohol be consumed in moderation only. Moderation is considered two drinks per day for men and one drink per day for women. One drink is defined as 12 ounces of beer, five ounces of wine, or 1.5 ounces of a distilled spirit.

Beware of Sugar and Alcohol

REMOVING OR CUTTING BACK ON SUGARS AND ALCOHOL
WILL EXPEDITE YOUR BODY COMPOSITION RESULTS.

Sugar is extremely addictive, and it can take two weeks
to break the habit.

Sugar disrupts the vitamin/mineral relationship in the body.

Sugar permanently changes the structure of your red blood
cells. It takes 90 days to create new, healthy red blood cells.

Avoid artificial sweeteners – they confuse your body's
metabolism and increase the body's toxic load burden.

Choose natural sweeteners whenever possible:
stevia, agave nectar, honey, molasses, and brown rice syrup.

Consume 12 grams or less of sugar in one sitting.

Daily Affirmation

I choose foods that provide me with naturally abundant energy.

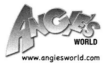

www.angiesworld.com

The Stress Factor

Two things are unavoidable in life: stress and taxes! In today's demanding lifestyle, we seem to feel like we need to take on more and more each day. We have become masters at multitasking and working until we collapse. It's an interesting phenomenon, since in today's age, we have more equipment and tools to help make our lives easier, yet we seem to be busier! We have washing machines, dishwashers, microwaves, cars, cell phones, computers, indoor plumbing, yet we don't have time to do anything. All this time racing the clock is making our lives more stressful.

Stress comes from many factors: environmental, physiological, metabolic, and psychological. Each factor contributes to an unhealthy, unbalanced life.

Stress is often the number one reason you can't release weight. When we are stressed, our bodies produce extra cortisol. Cortisol is a hormone produced by the adrenal cortex, which is a part of the adrenal gland. Your adrenal glands are located on top of each of your kidneys (they look like a little Hershey kiss on top of each kidney). Cortisol is commonly referred to as *the stress hormone* as it is involved in response to stress and anxiety. When we our under stress, the fight-or-flight response is triggered, which leads to the release of various hormones (including cortisol and adrenaline. *Fight or flight* means that either our body needs to attack an enemy via combat or we need to run like hell. If our body stays in this state for too long (i.e., chronic daily stress), our health becomes at risk.

When cortisol is overly active due to stress, it causes:
- hyperglycemia (high blood sugar), leading to mood swings and fatigue
- damage to memory receptors in the brain and impaired learning
- high blood pressure
- our body to hold onto extra-cellular water, making us feel bloated
- immune system function to decrease
- bone formation to decrease (thus favoring osteoporosis)
- weight gain (due to slowing of the metabolism)
- cravings for fatty, salty, and sugary foods
- metabolic syndrome (storing of abdominal fat, leading to many diseases)
- emotional eating, where you would eat more than you normally would

In normal release, cortisol helps:
- restore balance in the body after stress
- balance free amino acids in your blood
- keep potassium and copper levels balanced
- stimulate the liver to detoxify
- keep insulin in check to balance out glucose concentrations in the blood
- stimulate gastric secretion
- reduce inflammation
- keep you focused, energetic, and alert

Cortisol needs to be in perfect balance because an increase or reduction in cortisol can have negative effects in the body.
Factors that reduce cortisol levels include:
- magnesium supplementation
- essential fatty acids
- phosphatidylserine (also called PS) supplementation, which is derived from soy

- vitamin C
- black tea
- music therapy
- massage therapy
- laughing
- meditation

Most people have excess cortisol production in their bodies and would benefit greatly by taking the above measures to reduce their cortisol levels.

Factors that increase cortisol levels include:
- caffeine
- sleep deprivation
- intense or prolonged exercise
- hypoestrogenism
- melatonin supplementation
- burnout
- subcutaneous adipose tissue (fat that's directly under the skin)
- anorexia nervosa
- oral contraceptives in athletic women
- commuting (related to length of trip, the amount of effort involved and the predictability of the trip)

Environmental triggers of stress include:
- smog
- air pollution
- traffic exhaust
- cigarette smoke
- household cleaners
- insecticides and pesticides
- artificial sweeteners

Physiological triggers of stress include:
- accidents
- cuts and burns
- pain
- surgery
- prolonged or intense exercise
- poor sleep
- physical abuse
- illness

Metabolic triggers of stress include:
- oxidative stress
  (caused by incomplete breakdown of particles in the body)
- nutrient deficiency
- inflammation
- poor dietary habits

Psychological triggers of stress include:
- anxiety (a feeling of apprehension or fear)
- anger
- aggravation
- upset feelings
- temper tantrums
- emotional hurt
- mental abuse
- loneliness
- guilt

Stress can come from any situation and everybody's ability to deal with stress is quite different. In fact what may be stressful to one may not be stressful to another. Stress is a normal part of life, and in moderation, it can help motivate you to become more productive. It can help you perform better in an interview or presentation, increase your abilities in a sport or competition, or keep you focused when you have a major deadline at work. The stress response can save your life in an emergency, giving you lightning speed responses and super human strength. However, when stress is continuous, it can lead to poor health.

Signs of stress can be categorized into four areas: physical, cognitive, emotional, and behavioral.

Physical symptoms include:
- muscle tension
- sweating
- dry mouth
- headache
- brain fog
- twitching or shaking
- stomach ache or cramps
- rapid heart beat or irregular heartbeat
- chest tightness
- fatigue
- backaches
- diarrhea
- loss of sexual interest
- insomnia
- difficulty breathing

Cognitive symptoms include:
- difficulty concentrating
- forgetfulness
- worrying
- thoughts of death
- poor attention to detail
- perfectionist tendencies
- indecisiveness
- feeling helpless
- catastrophizing (blowing things out of proportion)

Emotional symptoms include:
- poor self-esteem
- suspiciousness
- guilt
- weeping
- loss of motivation
- moodiness
- depression

Behavioral symptoms include:
- increased alcohol use
- cigarette smoking
- increased caffeine use
- drug use
- violence
- overeating
- weight gain or loss
- relationship conflict
- decreased activity

Managing your stress is critical to obtaining a healthy, balanced body. Follow these guidelines to reduce stress in your life:
1. Eat a healthy diet:
   a. eating every 3-4 hours
   b. eating a variety of different foods
   c. eating in moderation
   d. making sure you are getting protein, carbohydrates, and good fats in each meal

2. Get a good night's sleep of 7- 8 ½ hours per night for adults and 8 – 9 ½ hours for children and teens

3. Exercise regularly:
    a. ideally, one hour per day, 6 days per week
    b. weight training at least 3 days per week
    c. cardiovascular exercise 6 days per week

4. Engage in at least one pleasurable activity each day:
    a. massage, yoga, stretching
    b. dreaming, meditating, relaxation techniques
    c. dancing
    d. laughing, being with friends
    e. listening to music
    f. exercise: walking, biking, sports, weight training
    g. artistic: painting, building, writing, being creative
    h. intimacy: kissing, hugging
    i. sexual intercourse

5. Use alcohol and caffeine in moderation:
    a. one drink per day for women
    b. two drinks per day for men

6. Set realistic goals:
    a. for yourself
    b. for your job
    c. your family
    d. short term (30, 60, 90 days)
    e. long term (1, 5, 10 years)

7. Develop a good support system:
    a. counseling
    b. accountability partner
    c. clubs, groups, and organizations
    d. religious participation
    e. family and friendships

8. Maintain a positive attitude:
  a. read motivational books
  b. attend inspirational events
  c. stop listening to/watching bad news
  d. avoid gossip and negative thinking
  e. watch motivating movies/shows

If you notice in the above outline on dealing with stress, the best option is action. As you ponder what action will best suit your lifestyle, let's dive into learning more about exercise.

The Stress Factor

STRESS IS OFTEN THE NUMBER ONE REASON
WE CAN'T RELEASE FAT.

Signs of stress can be categorized into four areas: physical, cognitive, emotional, and behavioral.

Guideline to reduce stress in your life:
1. Eat a healthy diet
2. Get a good night sleep
    7 – 8 ½ hours for adults,
    8 – 9 ½ hours for children and teens.
3. Exercise regularly –
    ideally for an hour each day, 6 days per week
4. Engage in one pleasurable activity each day
5. Use alcohol and caffeine in moderation
6. Set realistic goals
7. Develop a support system
8. Maintain a positive attitude

Daily Affirmation

I am strong mentally and physically.

I deserve time to play and engage in pleasurable activities.

When I manage my stress, I manage my weight!

I develop positive relationships with myself, my family, and my community.

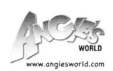

Move!

You've heard it before: If you don't use it, you lose it. And it's correct. This goes for your mind as well as your body. You have to move to be in optimal health. There are three main elements of fitness: strength training, cardiovascular exercise, and flexibility.

Strength training provides changes in your body composition. If you want to see your shape change, this is the fitness element for you. Think about this, every pound of muscle on your body will burn 2 ½ times more calories per day than fat burns! This means that by adding more muscle to your frame, you will turn your body into a calorie-eating furnace! Strength training is the reason I got excited about fitness. I love to eat and when I found out I could eat more AND still become leaner, I said, "Sign me up!" I was never one to starve myself or skip a meal, and I knew that this was the wrong way to release weight anyway. So when I discovered this secret about weight training I knew it was something I had to do.

Keep in mind, the opposite is also true: If you starve off muscle from your body, your body will burn 2 ½ times less calories per day! This is a scary thought!

Many diets on today's market do not focus on fat loss, they focus on weight loss. They do not test your body to see if you are losing muscle, fat, or water. In fact, they don't care. They guarantee *weight* loss, whatever that may be. Disturbingly enough, if you go to any of these fad weight-loss clinics, you will notice that most of the people who have reached their goal weight don't look very good. They look skinny-fat, not healthier and younger looking. When your body loses muscle instead of fat, your body composition worsens. Body composition is a ratio of fat to muscle; therefore, if you lose more muscle, you are essentially more fat. This fat isn't just underneath your skin making you not fit into your clothes. This fat is buried inside your organs, in your muscles, in your heart, lining your arteries and veins, and it is even stored inside your bone! Fat inside these areas leads to heart disease, high blood pressure, high cholesterol, high blood sugar levels, and lowered immune system function.

If you already have a weight problem and you do one of these fad diets, you not only put yourself at jeopardy for the above illnesses but you also risk becoming fatter!

For example, let's say you are a 180-pound person with one hundred pounds of fat-free mass on your body (Fat-free mass is everything on your body that is not fat: organs, muscles, connective tissues, bones). You would need 1700 calories per day to sustain the one hundred pounds of lean muscle. You are obviously eating more than 1700 calories since you are overweight. Now you put yourself on a fad diet and lose an additional ten pounds of lean muscle mass. At ninety pounds of lean muscle mass, you now need to consume only 1530 calories per day. After dieting, you will become *heavier* than before dieting. This is because you will go back to your old eating habits that were above 1700 calories, and you now only need 1530 calories.

When starting a weight training program (as with any new program), it is important to not do too much, too fast. As a personal trainer I have seen far too many people try to do everything they used to do in high school the very first day back in the gym after not exercising for over ten years. This is a recipe for disaster. Not only will they be tired and exhausted from the ordeal, they will most likely need to take the rest of the week off to recover. Remember consistency is the key. They won't be very consistent if they only show up at the gym once a week.

A myth about women who weight train is that they will become muscle-bound and look like a man. This is not true. Their fears are often confirmed by pictures found over the Internet of these manly women that would put The Incredible Hulk to shame. Women cannot look like men, unless they take male hormones, specifically testosterone. So you need not worry about this happening to you or your wife/girlfriend, unless steroids are in the picture.

Muscle builds at a very slow rate. The most new muscle a person can put on in a month is two pounds, and these two pounds will be spread over the entire body, not just in one area. Keep in mind that I said new muscle. Your muscular system has muscle memory. This means that even if you stop training for awhile, your body will remember how to put back that muscle when you start training, even if it's been twenty years. It is much easier for a person who used to be active or a post-athlete to get back into shape in their later years because of this fact. It is not uncommon for post-athletes to pack on ten pounds of muscle in just one month if they start to eat right and exercise again. This is because of the body's memory of this muscle mass. Often this muscle mass was still present in the body; it just wasn't metabolically active. Once stimulated, it re-activates itself. It is much harder for the person who has been sedentary his or her entire life to build muscle because it is new for the system. Don't get discouraged; it can be done! It will be at a rate of just two pounds per month. For men this seems like a disappointment but don't worry, you can pack on twenty-four pounds of solid muscle in one year and that will be impressive.

For women this is great, too, because it means that you can slowly watch the muscle appear on your body. If you feel you are getting too muscular in a particular area, you can change your workout and adjust your weights accordingly.

If you are serious about seeing changes in your physique, you will want to weight train three times per week, ideally, working different body parts each day. My recommendation follows:

Monday: Chest, biceps, and triceps

Wednesday: Legs

Friday: Shoulders and back

Abs can be worked out everyday, but ideally, you will want to do different exercises for them each day. For instance, on Monday when I work my chest, I will work my abs on a Swiss ball. I lie on top of the Swiss ball with the ball on my mid to low back, with my feet on the ground. I put dumbbells in my hands and will perform crunches while doing a chest press or fly. This will work my chest with my abs.

On Wednesday, after working my legs I will lie on the floor and perform leg lifts, again, incorporating the body part I am training for the day (legs) into my ab workout.

Finally on Friday, I like to use the Roman chair. This is where you hang on a machine using your upper body (shoulders) to keep you up while you perform leg raises and knee lifts. Another option would be to use a medicine ball, which would require shoulder strength.

If your abs are sore, make sure to give them twenty-four hours to recover.

When weight training, you must decide what you are trying to achieve before you start working out. Are you trying to tone and tighten, or are you trying to build muscle mass? The reason these questions are so important is because the answer will determine how many reps you will be performing in the gym. Reps are the amount of times you will repetitively do the action. If you said yes to toning and tightening, you will want to stick to lighter weights and perform 15 -20 reps at a time. One to two sets is ideal for toning and tightening. A set is the number of times you will perform the repetitive motion (reps).

If you answered yes to building mass, you will want to stick to six, eight, or ten reps with a heavier weight. The weight should be heavy enough where you will fatigue by the last rep, yet light enough to perform the exercise correctly throughout the reps.

If you find yourself swinging or using poor form, the weight is too heavy. When trying to build muscle, aim for three or four sets of any given exercise.

Ideally a typical workout should be an hour long. This includes thirty minutes of weight training and thirty minutes of cardio exercise.

If you are trying to release weight and tone and tighten, your cardio should be performed first. If you are trying to build muscle, cardio should be saved for last.

If you have achieved the body composition that you desire, it only takes twice a week to maintain it, provided you continue to eat clean. This will not take up too much of your time, but it will be well worth it.

When new to strength training, it would be ideal to hire a personal trainer to show you proper form and posture while training. Many injuries can be prevented by learning how to do things right the first time, and remember what I told you about muscle memory. If you teach yourself the wrong way to do an exercise, chances are you are going to repeat the bad habit over and over again. You will train your muscles into a faulty recruitment pattern. This can take months and even years to correct with a personal trainer.

I offer virtual training online for those who can't afford to hire one-on-one sessions with a personal trainer. Virtual training is offered at a fraction of the cost and allows you to see the exercise being performed correctly by watching a video. The program allows you to download and print the workout to take with you to the gym or wherever you decide to workout. Training programs are customized and can contain free weights, machines, elastic bands, cables, medicine balls, Swiss balls, body weight, or any combination of the above. Though there is really no substitute to one-on-one training, virtual training would be the next best thing.

Once reserved only for the rich and famous, personal training has reached the mainstream. Having the expertise of a personal trainer can accelerate your results in the gym and expand your knowledge of a healthy lifestyle. Having a personal trainer helps us to manage the most precious asset that we all possess and that is our health. Investing in a trainer is investing in yourself!

A good personal trainer can:
- assess your health and fitness status
- design a safe and appropriate exercise routine
- teach you the best way to exercise
- help you get MAXIMUM benefit from your gym time
- speed up your learning curve
- track your progress and tackle plateaus

- push you past your comfort level which is difficult to do on your own
- provide accountability, the hardest part of sticking with your nutrition and exercise plan
- keep you motivated

Your personal trainer will be your partner throughout your transformation!

Your best bet is to find a good personal trainer that has been accredited by a third party agency. This keeps the accreditation objective and well-rounded. Some of the most respected in the industry are the American College of Sports Medicine (ACSM), the National Strength and Conditioning Association (NSCA), the American Council on Exercise (ACE) and the International Sports Sciences Association (ISSA). Your trainer also needs to be certified in CPR/First Aid.

Be sure to ask about his or her experience with clients like you. So if you are hoping to improve your golf game, for instance, or if you are someone with a heart condition or arthritis, seek a trainer and organization with expertise and experience in those areas. Be prepared to answer specific questions about your goals and history.

Once you have picked your trainer and you are comfortable, listen to him or her and communicate. Your results will be directly related to a positive relationship with this person. Make sure to take advantage of the precious time you have with these professionals especially in regards to their wealth of knowledge. You can learn and apply this knowledge not only at the gym but to your lifestyle outside of the gym. Much of the information you obtain from a GREAT trainer can serve you well for much of your life as you constantly improve your overall health and well-being.

Please note that it may not be possible to train ALL the time with your trainer due to time or monetary concerns. Some clients work with their trainer once a week and are self-motivated enough to weight train themselves the other days. Others may check in with their trainer a couple of times per month and go it alone the other days. Many, however, like the dedicated appointment three times per week and find that it keeps them accountable and consistent. Pick what works best for you!

Muscle tends to disappear faster than it appears. Meaning, it takes just two weeks to lose muscle, the same muscle that took months to put back on. If you take a week off for vacation or due to illness, your muscle will be unaffected. But by the second week, you will have noticeable changes in your strength and composition. It's important to continue weight training while on vacation and business travel. If you are sick, taking a break is a good idea. The rule of thumb for exercise and weight training is this: If you are having symptoms below the neck, take the day off. If you are having symptoms from the neck up, it is safe to workout. If you decide to workout, make sure to listen to your body. Decreasing intensity and overall time in the gym is generally a good idea during this time.

Cardiovascular exercise refers to endurance exercises like running, swimming, biking, and aerobics. Just like the name implies, it provides benefits to your cardiovascular system. Cardio is a great tool to make you a smaller version of your current self. It will not provide muscular changes the way strength training will.

Any time you are performing an endurance exercise your body is rapidly burning up glycogen stores (remember the honey story). When stores are depleted, it is too difficult to convert fat as energy while you are exercising. Instead, your body will begin to burn up muscle tissue. This explains why marathon runners are extremely lean, weighing in on the emaciated side. Cyclists tend to be on the leaner side as well. But have you ever watched the Olympics and noted the difference between the sprinters and the marathoners? Wow. The sprinters are loaded with muscle. The sprinters perform short duration, high intensity work. We call this interval training in the gym.

Interval training is when you bring your heart rate up to its upper max limits for thirty to sixty seconds and then bring it back down to a lower training zone rate.

To determine your cardio training zone (60 -80% of your maximum heart rate), use this calculation:

Two hundred and twenty minus your age equals your maximum heart rate (220 – 40 yrs = 180MHR). 180 beats per minute is the maximum heart rate for a 40-year old person.

Then take that number and multiply it by .60 and .80.
(Ex. 180 x .60 = 108   and 180 x .80 = 144)
This will be your cardio training zone. In this example, 108-144 beats per minute.

In this example, this individual could perform interval exercises by walking at a speed where his/hers heart rate was at 108 for a minute, then sprinting or jogging so that his/hers heart rate is at 144 beats per minute for thirty seconds. Repeat this cycle at least five times.

Cardiovascular exercises can be performed six days a week, with one day off for complete rest. Variety is the spice of life, so try changing up your cardio exercises each day. If you are set on a particular cardio exercise, that's okay, too. Just make sure you vary your training each day. Choose a few shorter, higher intensity days, a few longer, lower intensity days, and perhaps one day of interval training.

Flexibility is a fitness element that is often neglected. Flexibility is described as the range of motion that is available to your joints. Flexibility reduces the chance of injury when playing a sport or in every day activities. Did you know that the average individual can expect to lose 70% of their flexibility from ages 20 -70?

Stretching is an excellent way to improve flexibility. A common misconception about stretching is that it is a waste of time. Because of this mindset, stretching exercises are often rushed through so fast that you don't get the benefit from each stretch. Or worse, they aren't performed at all. Lack of stretching leaves you vulnerable to connective tissue injuries, back pain, or muscle overuse. Muscles become shorter, tighter, and weaker if not stretched. Regular stretching not only can improve these problems, but it improves muscle balance around a joint, thus improving posture. It also increases the blood and nutrient supply to muscles and cartilage, thereby reducing muscle soreness. The best time to stretch is after physical labor or exercise, when the muscles are still warm, because it helps the body get rid of lactic acid and promotes the recovery of muscles.

Do not stretch on cold muscles! Warm up for at least at few minutes. Most people think that stretching is a warm-up before exercise or physical labor; it is not. A warm-up raises body temperature and increases blood flow to the muscles decreasing your chance for injury.

Think about this: If you were to put a rubber band inside the freezer and then pull it out and start stretching it, the rubber band would snap. This is much like how your muscles would react when stretched while cold. On the contrary, if you were to put the rubber band in the microwave for a few seconds, you would be able to stretch the rubber band easily, without breaking it.

When stretching, hold the stretch for twenty to sixty seconds. Hold the stretch at a mild point of tension, not to the point of pain. Never bounce while stretching! Instead, use your breath to help you stretch further. This can be done by inhaling in, and while exhaling pushing your body more into the stretched position.

While stretching is great for your body, there are times when stretching should be avoided. This would include:
- Following muscle strains or ligament sprains
- When joints or muscles are infected, inflamed or hurt
- After a recent fracture
- When sharp pains are felt in the joint or muscle.

Yoga and Pilates are other great avenues to pursue for flexibility. Yoga originated in India and originally was a philosophy, not a physical practice. Over time, it has incorporated breathing, stretching, and relaxation techniques. Not only is yoga fantastic for flexibility, it increases lubrication of the joints, ligaments and tendons. It also massages all the organs of the body. According to www.healthandyoga.com, "Yoga is perhaps the only form of activity which massages all the internal glands and organs of the body in a thorough manner, including those, such as the prostate, that hardly get externally stimulated during our entire lifetime. Yoga acts in a wholesome manner on the various body parts. This stimulation and massage of the organs in turn benefits us by keeping away disease and providing a forewarning at the first possible instance of a likely onset of disease or disorder."

Pilates (puh-LAH-teez) was designed by Joseph Pilates not only to improve flexibility, but to strengthen the body's core, mobilize the spine, and improve body awareness. Pilates can be done on a mat with a system of floor exercises or with a reformer. A reformer is an apparatus that Joseph Pilates designed himself to assist the body in a variety of movement.

When starting up an exercise program, you may want to chose one modality at a time, either cardiovascular, strength or flexibility exercises. But ideally, you will want to incorporate all three into your workout routine.

Based on Chinese medicine, it is best to work out for less strenuous, longer durations of time in the spring and summer and for more intense, shorter workouts in the fall and winter.

Another benefit from movement is that it is nature's way of detoxifying your body.

Unlike your circulatory system where you have a heart pumping your blood throughout your body, your lymphatic system relies on movement to circulate it.

Because your lymphatic system doesn't have a pump, it is imperative that you move to move your lymph. Your lymphatic system contains many components of your immune system and if you are sedentary, it will become toxic from being stagnant.

Wrap-up

Move

INCORPORATE ALL THREE MAIN ELEMENTS OF FITNESS:

    STRENGTH TRAINING

    CARDIOVASCULAR EXERCISE

    FLEXIBILITY

Every pound of muscle on your body burns 2 1/2 times as many calories as fat per day. Ideally weight train 3 times per week and perform cardio 6 days per week (30 min).

To determine your cardio training zone:
    220 - your age = Maximum heart rate (MHR)
    Take MHR and times by .6 and by .8
    This will determine your training zone (60 -80% of MHR)

Use proper form and if possible, seek the advice of a personal trainer and/or nutritionist.

Flexibility is a critical element to fitness. Do not stretch on cold muscles!

When stretching, hold the stretch for 20 – 60 seconds.
Hold the stretch at a mild point of tension, not to the point of pain.

Yoga and Pilates are great avenues for flexibility.

Daily Affirmation

I choose exercise that I enjoy to improve my body AND my mind.

Exercise is an investment that benefits me and my family.

My lean body has abundant energy.

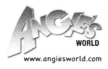

WORLD

Detoxification

The art of cleansing our bodies has been around for thousands of years. The use of herbs and vegetables to treat diseases began in our earliest civilizations. Records on Egyptian papyrus describe potions used to treat various illnesses, most of which were derived from vegetable substances. Hindu and Greek medicine used many vegetable derivatives as well. Many of the chemicals found in these vegetable derivatives are still in use in modern medicine. In India a system of traditional medicine using complementary and alternative medicine is used. It is called Ayurveda. It employs the use of lifestyle management, herbs, massage, and yoga.

Many companies (often funded by the pharmaceutical companies) spend considerable energy trying to convince us that it is a waste of time and money to detoxify the body. They claim that detoxification products do not work and that our bodies are fully capable of naturally detoxifying anything that is foreign or toxic to the body.

If this is so, why is it that when you take a look around, the majority of our population (69% of the U.S. population is overweight, and 35% are obese) is not able to rid their bodies of extra body fat? Remember, we store our toxins in our fat cells. The more toxic we are, the more fat cells we produce to store toxic load.

Other common signs of toxic burden are inflammation (puffiness), water weight (edema), bags under the eyes, headaches, muscular aches and pains, and fatigue. The most common sites where we store water weight in relation to toxic load are the areas in which we have the greatest amount of lymph nodes; for example, underneath the chin, around the neck, under our armpits and back of upper arms, around the inner thigh, and behind the knees. If these areas feel like a water balloon to the touch, then you are experiencing a toxic burden in your body. Extensive research shows that it is not a question of if we are carrying a burden of these toxins, but rather how much and to what extent they affect our health.

In fact, if it were true that we could safely remove all toxins from our body then poisoning would not be fatal to our bodies. Our bodies would naturally speed up the detoxification process to eliminate the poison, thus, avoiding death. Poisoning has been around since 4500 BC. It was used as a weapon for assassination by every social class, even nobility, to dispose of unwanted political or economic opponents.

If you consider all the evidence, it is obvious that our bodies can't totally eliminate toxic loads naturally or keep up with the toxic burden we are throwing on them, and they really could use our help.

Your body can tolerate a certain level of toxin load. For each person this tolerance level will be different depending on many factors. They include your exposure levels, your lifestyle, diet, drug intake, general habits, medical treatments, surrounding environment, the strength and clear functioning of your faculties of elimination and the general strength of your immune system. There is a direct correlation between toxic load and disease in the body:

- Immunological toxicity may be a factor in the development of asthma, allergies, skin disorders, chronic infections, and cancer.
- Neurological toxicity affects cognition, mood, and overall mental functioning.
- Endocrine toxicity affects reproduction, menstruation, libido, metabolic rate, stress tolerance, glucose regulation, and more.

Did you know (according to the U.S. Environment Protection Agency):

- More than 4 billion pounds of chemicals were released into the ground in 2000, threatening our natural ground water sources.
- Over 260 million pounds of chemicals were discharged into-

surface waters (i.e., lakes, rivers, and oceans).

- Nearly 2 billion pounds of air emissions were pumped into the atmosphere.
- Several thousand food additives are intentionally added to our food supply, and thousands more slip into our food supply unintentionally during harvesting, processing, or packaging. In fact, the average American consumes about124 pounds of food additives a year!
- Over 400 pesticides and herbicides are currently licensed for use on food crops, and every year over 2.5 billion pounds are dumped on crop lands, forests, lawns, and fields.

Your exposure to toxins is increased in the following common ways:

- eating a diet high in processed foods and fat
- drinking tap water
- excessive consumption of caffeinated beverages
- excessive alcohol consumption
- smoking, including second hand smoke
- recreational drug use
- chronic use of medication(s)
- consumption of artificial sweeteners, food colors, and dyes
- eating the same vegetables and fruits each day
- air pollution: smog
- cooking with Teflon pots and pans
- eating at restaurants that use MSG and other flavor-enhancers
- lack of strenuous exercise
- liver dysfunction
- kidney problems
- intestinal dysfunction
- occupational exposure
- using pesticides, herbicides, paint, and other toxic substances without adequate protective gear
- living or working near areas of high vehicle traffic or industrial plants

To determine how toxic the environment you live in is, go to http://www.scorecard.org. When investigating my area (Riverside County, California), it ranked among the dirtier 30% of all counties in the U.S. in terms of ozone depleting potential. This website also provides a list of the top polluting companies in your community as well as the major pollutants (chemicals) in your environment. For Riverside County, the top five major chemicals we are exposed to are N-Butyl Alcohol (81.908 pounds), Glycol ethers (74,405 pounds), 1,1Dichloro-1-fluoroethane (67,803 pounds), Toluene (30,629 pounds), and Nitrate compounds (29,308 pounds).

TOP 5 CHEMICALS IN RIVERSIDE COUNTY & THEIR SUSPECTED TOXICITY

	N-Butyl Alcohol	Glycol ethers	1,1Dichloro-1-fluoroethane	Toluene	Nitrate compounds
Cardiovascular or blood toxicant	X	X	X	X	X
Gastrointestinal or liver toxicant	X	X		X	
Kidney toxicant		X		X	
Neurotoxicant	X	X	X	X	
Reproductive toxicant				X	
Skin or Sense organ toxicant	X				
Respiratory toxicant	X	X			
Developmental toxicant		X		X*	
Immunotoxicant				X	

*Toluene is a recognized developmental toxicant

92

My county's water quality ranking was also above the national average in terms of dirtiest/worst.

As bad as this may seem, in 2004 Riverside County ranked among the cleanest/best 20% of all counties in the U.S. in terms of the number of designated Superfund sites. A Superfund site is any land in the U.S. that has been contaminated by hazardous waste and identified by the Environmental Protection Agency (EPA) as a candidate for cleanup because it poses a risk to human health or the environment or both. There are only three Superfund sites in Riverside County: Alark Hard Chrome, March Air Reserve Base, and Stringfellow.

Conditions at Proposal (July 27, 2000): The Alark Hard Chrome site occupies approximately 0.25 acre in a light industrial area of the city of Riverside. An electroplating shop operated on site from 1971 to 1985. Eighteen open plating tanks were housed in the front and middle rooms of the shop. The tanks were set directly on the ground in cut-outs in the concrete floor. As metal parts were lifted out of each tank, the plating solution would drip and spill onto the floor and into the three to five-inch gap between the tank and the floor. Plating solutions were also allegedly discharged directly into a four -foot wide by forty-foot deep pit located in the middle room. Water from washdowns in the plating areas flowed into three floor drains that were routed to a five hundred gallon underground holding tank located outside the rear of the building. The back room of the shop housed grinders and polishers. During a 1982 investigation of the site, personnel from the Riverside County Department of Health observed "pools of chemicals" outside the back door of the shop. In 1985, the owners of Alark Hard Chrome ceased operations and took the plating tanks off site. The underground holding tank was also taken off site sometime in the middle or late 1980s.

With all this environmental exposure, you might realize that detoxification is necessary primarily due to what we are unknowingly inhaling. Add to these staggering numbers what we choose to ingest into our bodies: artificial chemicals, hydrogenated fats, excitotoxins, cigarette smoke, alcohol, preservatives, and food colorings/dyes.

ARE YOU TOXIC? TAKE THE TEST

Rate each of the following symptoms based upon your health profile for the past 30 days:

POINT SCALE:

0 = NEVER OR ALMOST NEVER have the symptom

1 = OCCASIONALLY have it, effect is NOT SEVERE

2 = OCCASIONALLY have it, effect is SEVERE

3 = FREQUENTLY have it, effect is NOT SEVERE

4 = FREQUENTLY have it, effect is SEVERE

(Add up the numbers to arrive at a total for each section, and then add the totals for each section to arrive at the grand total.)

DIGESTIVE SYSTEM

_____ Nausea or vomiting

_____ Diarrhea

_____ Constipation

_____ Belching, passing gas

_____ Bloated feeling

_____ Heartburn

_____ TOTAL

EARS

_____ Itchy ears

_____ Earaches, ear infections

_____ Drainage from ears

_____ Ringing in ears

_____ Hearing loss

_____ TOTAL

EMOTIONS

_____ Mood swings

_____ Anxiety, fear, nervousness

_____ Anger, irritability

_____ Depression

_____ TOTAL

ENERGY/ACTIVITY

_____ Fatigue, Sluggishness

_____ Apathy, lethargy

HEART

_____ Skipped heartbeats

_____ Rapid heartbeats

_____ Chest pain

_____ TOTAL

JOINT/MUSCLES

_____ Pain or aches in joints

_____ Arthritis

_____Stiffness, limited movement

_____ Pain, aches in muscles

_____ Weakness or tiredness in joints

_____ TOTAL

LUNGS

_____ Chest Congestion

_____ Asthma, bronchitis

_____ Shortness of breath

_____ Difficulty breathing

_____ TOTAL

MIND

_____ Poor memory

_____ Confusion

_____ Poor concentration

_____ Poor coordination

_____ Difficulty making decisions

ENERGY/ACTIVITY *(continued)*
_____ Hyperactivity
_____ Restlessness
_____ TOTAL

EYES
_____ Watery, itchy eyes
_____ Swollen, reddened, or sticky eyelids
_____ Dark circles under eyes
_____ Blurred/tunnel vision
_____ TOTAL

HEAD
_____ Headaches

_____ Faintness
_____ Dizziness
_____ Insomnia
_____ TOTAL

NOSE
_____ Stuffy nose
_____ Sinus problems
_____ Hay fever
_____ Sneezing attacks
_____ Excessive mucus
_____ TOTAL

SKIN
_____ Acne
_____ Genital itch, discharge
_____ Hives, rashes, dry skin
_____ Hair loss
_____ Flushing or hot flashes
_____ Excessive sweating
_____ TOTAL

MIND *(continued)*
_____ Stuttering, stammering
_____ Slurred speech
_____ Learning disabilities
_____ TOTAL

MOUTH/THROAT
_____ Chronic coughing
_____ Gagging, frequent need to clear throat
_____ Sore throat, hoarse
_____ Swollen or discolored tongue, gums, or lips
_____ Canker sores
_____ TOTAL

WEIGHT
_____ Binge-eating/drinking
_____ Craving certain foods
_____ Excessive weight
_____ Compulsive eating
_____ Water retention
_____ Underweight
_____ TOTAL

OTHER
_____ Frequent illness
_____ Frequent or urgent need to urinate
_____ TOTAL

GRAND TOTAL _____

KEY:

50 or higher
High level of general symptoms indicates symptoms of elevated toxic load. It is recommended that you see a certified nutritionist to aid you in a detoxification diet protocol. Ideally use a 28-day elimination diet.

15 – 49
Moderate level of general symptoms indicates moderate symptoms of toxic load. Please see a certified nutritionist for a 10-day elimination diet.

14 or less
Low level of general symptoms indicates minimal indicators of toxic load. An elimination diet is not needed.

When deciding to detoxify your body, make sure to buy a product that supports BOTH Phase I and Phase II activities of the liver by providing key ingredients such as L-glutathione, N-acetylcysteine, taurine, sodium sulfate, and catechins from green tea. If needed, alkalizing factors such as potassium citrate can be included to enhance toxin excretion.

There are many detox products that can be purchased over the counter. Make sure you are buying from a reputable company that has a proven track record. Ideally you want to make sure the product is clinically tested and is backed by published research that shows it helps relieve symptoms and conditions associated with toxicity.

These anti-detox companies are right when they say most products on the market are a waste of money especially those made from synthetic ingredients or those only supporting phase I detoxification. Phase I detoxification is the first process of the liver to break a toxin down into an intermediate form so that it can be transformed into a water soluble molecule by the liver via phase II. This water-soluble molecule then can easily be removed via the kidneys. Without phase II, your body is actually in a more catastrophic state. These intermediate forms act much like free radicals. Free radical damage can lead to disease faster than any toxic burden. Your body needs to be supported throughout the detoxification process. In fact some people require additional support of phase III detoxification, which is the final process of removing the water-soluble toxins from your kidneys.

Whatever you decide to do, do not fast for detoxification purposes! Fasting does not support detoxification because it does not give the body the nutrients it needs to eliminate the toxic burden. The practice of fasting is more of a spiritual ritual than for detoxification purposes.

This spiritual detoxification technique was an ancient practice of Hinduism. They would set aside certain days of the year for women to fast and other days for men. It can still be observed in certain parts of India today, where they abstain from food and drink on the eleventh and twelfth days of every Hindu month. The ancient scriptures of Persia advocated fasting for spiritual purification. Yom Kippur, a sacred Jewish holiday, is also known as the Day of Atonement. It is believed that to fast on Yom Kippur is to emulate the angels in heaven, who do not eat or drink.

Some Christians and Catholics also observe a semi-fast during Lent, where they abstain from eating meat on Fridays.

Muslims observe an annual fast during the month of Ramadan. For an entire month, Muslims do not eat, drink, smoke, or have sex between sunrise and sundown. It is described in the Quran thus: "So that you may attain taqwa or God-consciousness."

Also, do not start a detox program when you are ill or feeling sick. Doing so will put an extra burden on your liver, kidneys, and lungs.

The Detoxification Process

Detoxification is a process by which your body transforms toxins into harmless molecules that can be excreted. This process takes place primarily in the liver and to a lesser degree in other tissues.

Detoxification is largely accomplished in 3 stages:

Phase I:
Certain enzymes change toxins into intermediate compounds

Phase II:
Other enzymes convert intermediate compounds into water-soluble molecules

Phase III:
Water-soluble molecules are excreted mainly via urine or bile/feces

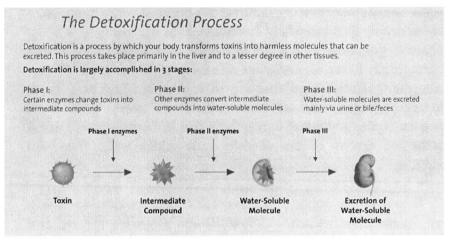

If our bodies don't accumulate toxins, then why is it that after a proper detox is performed, the symptoms from the above toxic test are reduced or completely eliminated? And why is it that ever since chemical companies started adding food additives, pesticides, man-made chemicals, and other non-organic substances that nature never intended for us to ingest, we have seen an increase in illness and disease such as cancer, heart disease, diabetes and obesity? Also we now have more prevalent neurological disorders such as depression, anxiety, attention deficit disorder, Alzheimer's disease, Lou Gehrig's disease, Multiple Sclerosis, and Autism.

Why is it that countries that still have whole-food-based diets have a fraction of these diseases? Why is it that when such countries adopt our Western diet, they begin to have these same diseases?

Detoxification should be an important part of your yearly health maintenance program, much like taking your yearly physical exam. Ideally, detoxification should be performed in the spring. This is when your body is most ready to remove toxins from your body. This theory goes along with Chinese medicine, where your body requires different foods and different exercises and intensities throughout the year. Conversely, detoxing in the winter is the hardest time for your body. This is the time when your body is in a more dormant state. However, detoxing <u>can</u> be done in the wintertime, specifically when an individual is under severe stress due to toxic burden. The body will be willing to remove these toxins immediately, regardless of what time of year it is. For optimum results, however, spring is the best time of year to perform a detox.

Just like anything in life, everything in moderation. Do not do more than two detoxification cleanses in one year. They are very hard on your system and more than two per year are not necessary, except under certain circumstances, which should be evaluated by a certified nutritionist or naturopathic doctor. A detox can be performed in as little as five days and can be continued up to thirty days, depending on toxicity. When performing a detox, it is important to seek advice from a certified, licensed nutritionist or naturopathic doctor. A professional will be able to safely determine which detox program is right for you. It is also important to realize that weekly detox products are not quick fixes and that a detox can not undo a bad eating lifestyle carried out 365 days of the year.

Detoxification

Detoxification should be an important part of your yearly health maintenance program, much like taking your yearly physical exam.

Exercise and water help the body to naturally eliminate toxins.

Use reputable supplements and the help of a nutritionist or naturopathic doctor to assist you during a true detox program.

Detoxing cleanses your body and your mind.

Daily Affirmation

Environmental toxins are inevitable, but my healthy choices in food and activities help to reduce their impact on me.

My choices support my body and it's natural detoxing processes.

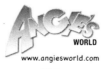

Accountability

Now that you have a strong foundation about what it takes to be healthy, it is important that you share your goals with your friends and family. Being accountable is a major factor of whether or not you will attain your goals. Ask your family to help you stay strong during your transformation. This means they will need to agree to not try to tempt you with bad food choices, not to put you in positions where you are likely to cave on your plan, and mostly, to help keep you honest and stick to your word. They can be there to remind you how important it is for you to exercise or choose a healthier meal when eating out.

When looking for accountability, it is important to surround yourself with others who are like-minded: those who are trying to change for the better, those who have already made the change, or those who are professionals in the field of change.

Having a friend or neighbor follow your same plan is a great way to stay on top of your goals. Depending on your needs or how self-motivated you are, you may need to see your accountability partner everyday or just once a week.

Becoming accountable to someone who has already achieved his or her own health goals is an excellent way to stay focused. This is a person who will have first-hand experience with what you are going through and will be able to share stories with you about frustrations, joys, and ultimate successes.

Hiring a professional to help you will ultimately fast-forward your results whether it be a lifestyle coach, a personal trainer, licensed nutritionist, or someone else in the field of wellness.

The first step to being accountable is to know what your goals are. You really want to write these down! Write them in a journal or on a sheet of paper that you can easily reference each day.

Write down your weekly goals, monthly goals, three-month goals, six-month goals, nine-month goals, and yearly goals. Write down every thought that comes to mind, no matter how big or small. Make sure you have realistic goals though. It's okay to dream big but writing down that you are going to release twenty pounds in one month is neither realistic nor healthy. A healthy weight loss rate is about three pounds a week or less. When first switching your diet from fast food to clean eating, it isn't uncommon for a person to drop ten pounds in the first week. This is due to water weight from the inflammation your body was holding onto from eating poorly. But once your eating plan is in full swing, strive for three pounds a week.

Perhaps you can write down small dietary changes per week, such as the following:

Week 1 and 2:
Stop drinking soda (regular or diet) and switch to
iced tea or water.
Week 3 and 4: Avoid cookies and other sugary snacks.
Week 5 and beyond:
Avoiding soda as well as sugary foods.

By slowly making new dietary choices, it becomes easier to stick to your new goals because you are not trying to completely change overnight.

Write out your detailed weekly and monthly goals and then make a copy. Give a copy to your accountability partner so he or she is aware of your goals.

I would also like to suggest a weekly accountability chart. This chart is filled out each week and given to your partner or is used as a tool to self check your progress.

An accountability chart should contain the following information:

WEEKLY ACCOUNTABILITY

Week _____ _____ Exact dates

Rate your week: ____ On a scale of 1 -10; 1 being lousy, 10 being amazing

What did you accomplish this week: _____

_____

_____

_____

Record weekly exercise here: What, how much/type, duration

Ex. Monday – bike ride, ten miles, forty-five minutes

Tuesday – weight training, shoulders and back, thirty minutes

You can even record total calories burned if you use a heart monitor.

What do I weigh at the end of the week? _____

You only need to record your weight once a week; it is not necessary to weigh everyday. Weigh in on the same day at approximately the same time. You can also record other information like caliper readings:

Arm: _____ Pelvic: _____ Glute: _____

If you have a scale that tells body fat percentage or other information, write it down too.

What do I feel really good about this week?

_____

_____

_____

Write down accomplishments you made in the gym such as adding more weight, doing more reps or increases in cardio performances, as well as how you are feeling, or how your clothes are fitting.)

What do I expect to accomplish next week?

_____

_____

Write down your intentions for the upcoming week.

What struggles/pitfalls am I encountering?

_____

_____

_____

Write down any challenges you are experiencing

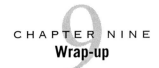

Accountability

Write down your goals.

Share your goals with your family and friends.

Find an accountability partner, someone who shares the same goals or has achieved successes with his/her health and lifestyle improvements.

Staying consistent is the key to success.

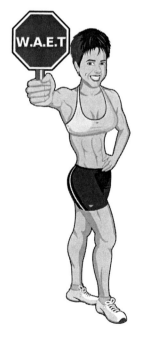

Daily Affirmation

*I continue to make positive
changes everyday.*

*I share my successes to reinforce
my own goals and to help those
around me with theirs.*

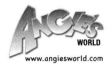

Starting your Lifestyle Change

When contemplating a lifestyle change, it is important to listen to your body and make sure the choices you are making are right for you. Only you truly know your body and know when it feels good or bad. Pushing yourself too hard or being too strict on yourself is not going to make lasting positive results.

If at any time you feel my suggestions are not right for you, make a change so that they do feel right. Make an appointment with a health care practitioner in your area to determine what your body needs specifically. You can log on to www.stopchronicdisease.com to find a therapeutic lifestyle change (TLC) nutritionist or practitioner.

If your goal is weight release, remember that you didn't put on the weight overnight, so you can't expect to release it that fast. Realistically you should only release three pounds per week.

If your goal is to build more muscle, remember that you can only put on two pounds of new muscle in a month. In order to do that you must eat right and rest your muscles in between workouts.

A true lifestyle change occurs when an action is consistently being performed, the key word being consistent. Starting and stopping a plan is not *consistent*. It is really important that you choose reasonable goals that can be followed through. Only then should you re-access your goals and perhaps increase your activity level or add another dietary change.

You will find that the fastest and easiest plan will not help make permanent changes. There are many fad diets out there that can make you drop ten pounds overnight. But remember that most of these diets will have you losing water weight and muscle. True fat loss takes a bit of time but leads to permanent changes over time. When you are ready to stop yo-yo dieting, a therapeutic lifestyle change is ultimately what you are looking for.

Some key questions you should ask yourself when trying a new program, whether it be exercise or a new eating plan, are:

1. Does this feel balanced?

> A healthy eating plan will contain all the major macronutrients: carbohydrates, proteins, and fats. It will not completely eliminate a major food group.

> A balanced workout program will contain weight training, cardiovascular exercise, and flexibility or stretching.

2. Can I maintain this program for the long term?

> If a plan feels like it is too much, too strict, or too limiting, you most likely will not make it a lifestyle, nor would you want to!

3. Do you feel healthier?

> A therapeutic lifestyle plan should provide you with adequate energy throughout the day. You should feel stronger, mentally more clear, and able to go through your day without crashing from low energy. You will no longer need to rely on caffeine or other energy drinks and pills to get through your day.

Keep in mind, a detox diet, which is a temporary plan, may initially decrease your energy due to your body's extensive internal cleansing.

Once you have achieved your goal weight, it is important to still maintain your program. You may need to adjust your calories slightly, depending on whether you were trying to release fat or gain muscle.

Earlier in this book I suggested that you only eat fruits and vegetables grown locally. This is the best way to help your body in the environment in which you are living. It also helps your environment by decreasing the amount of biofuels used to transport food across the planet. However, there are a few foods worth considering that may not grow in your area. They are called super foods. These are foods that are extremely high in antioxidants, vitamins, and minerals. These foods may or may not grow locally for you but are worth adding into a daily regimen.

Here is a brief list of super foods you may want to consider: goji berries (also known as wolf berries), hemp seeds, cacao, maca, cama cama, salmon, broccoli, sweet potatoes, berries, nuts, beans, kiwis, quinoa, barley, eggs, apricots, blueberries, peanut butter, cinnamon, pomegranate, yogurt, oats, avocado, acai, hot peppers, sprouts, apples, extra virgin olive oil, and green tea. There are more, but this is enough to get you started.

The more exotic super foods cost more and come with a larger carbon footprint because of the CO_2 produced by their journey to your grocery store.

Supporters of exotic super foods will remind you that these foods have higher ORAC values. ORAC stands for Oxygen Radical Absorbance Capacity, which is a fancy term describing the method used to measure the antioxidant power of a certain food.

There is a lot of talk in the marketplace in regards to which foods have the highest ORAC values. This is obviously done from a marketing standpoint to sell more of a certain super food.

All foods have an ORAC value. The higher the number, the better it is for you. However, ORAC numbers are often published in misleading ways. The USDA publishes ORAC numbers by a standard food serving of 100 grams. Goji berries, for instance, come in around 25,000 per 100 grams (Brunswick Labs). So the per gram ORAC value of goji berries is only 250. So when someone shows you an ORAC score, make sure you're comparing grams to grams. Most companies throw an ORAC number per serving, or per bottle, and sometimes, per nothing. Furthermore, it is extremely difficult to make direct comparisons between foods. Many factors can change the ORAC value reading by several thousand percent including harvest times, growing conditions, and physical state when tested (dried, fresh, freeze dried, concentrated extract). Dried samples tend to concentrate the antioxidant compounds.

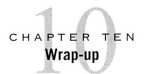

Starting My Lifestyle Change

Get to know your own body for lasting, long term results.

Lifestyle changes occur when my actions are consistently performed.

Daily Affirmation

My new lifestyle is a process that
I support with healthy and
positive choices everyday.

My life is balanced.

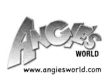

www.angiesworld.com

Final Thoughts

No matter where you start your journey toward wellness, it is a road worth traveling. When looking at life, it is not the quantity of years you live but the quality of those years. After all, what is the point of living to one hundred if the last twenty years you are bed ridden without the will to live because your body is in so much pain or filled with disease? I would much rather live a healthy, fulfilled life, doing everything my heart desires, and die when my body is tired, not when it is broken down.

When you realize how important it is to eat in a healthy way, you will realize that your body is capable of doing just about anything, providing you fuel it properly. You wouldn't put 87-octane gas in a custom car that runs only on premium. Your body is a custom car; treat it right and it will run smoothly and effortlessly.

I once heard a story about longevity. It had to do with whether a Ferrari or a Volkswagen Beetle would last longer. One might think that a Ferrari with its sleek style and state-of-the-art technology would outlast any Beetle. A Beetle is not made with such precision and obviously runs much more slowly. But perhaps the person with the Ferrari knows that he can run the Ferrari fast and take corners at 80 mph. The Ferrari can do this and may not even sputter a single time while its owner aggressively changes gears and puts his pedal to the metal. The owner of the Beetle, on the other hand, knows his car is not so finely constructed. He will drive it slower, making sure the oil is changed regularly as well as adhering to the recommended tune-ups. It is no surprise to predict that the Beetle will outlast the Ferrari under these circumstances.

In many a counseling session have I heard the words, "I don't have good genetics." Keep in mind what I have already taught you:

It's 80% nutrition, 10% working out, and 10% genetics. Regardless if you were born a sleek, high-performance body style or a soft, under-muscled design, it's what you make of your body and how you take care of it that will determine your longevity.

Think about playing a video game. Would you choose a heavy-set character to perform the tasks of jumping, kicking, running and fighting to the finish line? Or would you choose an athletic character? It's a no-brainer that the athletic character would have an easier time conquering the levels of the game. So why is it that we choose a heavier set character to live our game of life?

I have a client who is a chiropractor. He wanted to release weight because his blood pressure was out of control. Not only did he release the weight, he became a better chiropractor! How? He did manual adjustments on his clients' spine by pushing down on their backs with his hands. When he released his belly fat, he was able to get closer to his clients, making it easier for him to adjust his patients.

Many a client will come to see me complaining about lower back pain. This is often due to excessive belly fat. This forces their lumbar spine to arch excessively due to the extra load they are carrying. What area or areas of your body are in chronic pain? Wouldn't you give just anything to get rid of that pain for good? The answer may not be what you want to hear—get rid of the bad foods and drinks you are ingesting.

Every small choice you make to eliminate or stop a bad habit will be one step toward the path of health. The easiest way to accomplish this is to ask yourself, "Is this good for my body and soul?" If the answer is no, stay away.

My road to health is a continuous journey. I did not make all my changes overnight. Despite releasing weight and transforming my body in three months, I did not master health in those few months. At that time I still had some bad health habits, such as consuming artificial sweeteners and diet sodas. What I did at that time was take a little bit of information and make a lot of physical changes. We all know some way of releasing weight, most of the time we know it is the wrong way or, at least, not the healthiest way. Perhaps we take this road to jump start the process, but ultimately we know we have to make long term health changes to see lasting results. Once I understood why I was making these changes (not just to look good, but to fully and truly be healthy), I realized my journey had just begun.

Much like planning a vacation to Hawaii, you will have to make plans to make that vacation a reality. No matter how badly you want to go to Hawaii, you won't one day wake up and magically be there. You have to plan it. You have to call the travel agent and decide what week you want to go. You have to save up the money, call the airline, and make a hotel reservation. Once all the planning is done, you have to take action by driving yourself to the airport, flying on a plane, and taking a cab to the hotel. All these steps are critical to achieving your goal of being on vacation. Changing your body composition is no different. You can read hundreds of books and magazines on how to slim down or build muscle, and you can fantasize about what you would do once you have that dream body, but ultimately you have to make a plan and take action.

On my journey I would make dietary changes that I knew I could follow. Once they became habit, I would add more changes. I read all the books on nutrition I could get my hands on. It didn't take long to understand how bad artificial sweeteners were for my body. Once I knew that truth, I implemented a *no-artificial-sweetener rule* into my program. What I immediately realized was that I felt less hungry once I removed them from my diet. Turns out the amino acid L-phenylalanine is responsible for curbing your appetite when consumed in low dosages. However when consumed in higher amounts, it makes you feel hungrier! Yikes! Part of my ferocious appetite was chemically induced!

Farther along on my journey, I discovered how damaging genetically modified foods are for the body. The truth is they are bad for the planet! Recently an article was published about how the honey bees are dying and scientists couldn't find out why. Upon further investigation, they found a link to genetically modified foods. The modified foods did something to the pollen that caused the bees to die. In fact this problem has become so wide spread that farmers are now having to buy truckloads of bees to pollinate their crops. Every season they must buy again, even if their crops are not genetically modified. The reason is that bees travel very far to get pollen. They will go to other farms where genetically modified foods may be growing. Once this happens, the bees will die off. One blueberry farmer spent $70,000 a year to buy bees because of this problem. My question to you is this: If genetically modified foods can kill off entire bee populations, what are these foods doing to us at a cellular level? The articles that I read on this subject say that if honey bees become extinct, the only crops we will have on this planet will be wheat, soy, and corn because they are wind-pollinating, and do not rely on bees. Scarier than that is the fact that most people have food sensitivities to these foods! They are not well tolerated and often cause inflammatory responses in people.

With each passing year, more and more studies will come out that will give us new insight into why eating chemical ridden, processed food is bad for us. And as we learn more it becomes increasingly apparent that we need to go back to the basics and eat whole foods. Whole foods are foods that are minimally processed once they are harvested. Shopping the perimeter of a grocery store will provide you with all the whole foods you will need—vegetables, fruits, meats, and some dairy. Everything in the aisles should be avoided.

Ultimately what will be needed to achieve our health goals is a positive attitude and a willingness to be open about our food sources and choices. As we learn that caged animals produce stress hormones that get translated into our body as such, we will need to allow for free range farming. As we discover that growth hormones and antibiotics in our meats are causing our children to develop and mature at younger ages, we will need to find other ways to keep our cattle healthy. When we become aware of reverse osmosis water leeching our own minerals from our bones because it lacks its own minerals that are needed for absorption, we must rediscover natural water sources that are intended for our bodies.

The journey of health never truly ends. Our health and the health of future generations are dependent on our eagerness to learn and our passion toward healing ourselves and our planet. After all, if our planet is sick, so are we. Our struggle doesn't come from fighting off insects and diseases. Our journey becomes complete when we realize we need to co-exist in harmony with all creations. We must question trying to control our soils, the temperatures we grow foods, the insects that linger on our food supplies, how big our cattle will get, how many cattle will be produced, how much yield a crop will bear, and what plants should be allowed to live while others must die. It is when we let go of this control that we will achieve balance in our lives.

We have to start paying attention when we hear that Monsanto is buying out our seed banks. Monsanto owns the powerful weed killer called Round-up. Its main purpose in buying our seed banks is to test and genetically modify every living plant on our planet so that no other weed killer works except their product. Our seed banks were built so that in case of a nuclear attack or other unforeseen incidence where our food was no longer edible, we could go back and retrieve seeds that had not been affected from a world-wide devastation. What good will these seeds be if they are all genetically modified? Life as we know it will cease to exist.

After all how can we truly live balanced lives when everything in our environment is being controlled in a certain direction? How will we know our bodies' ideal weights when we are constantly ingesting chemicals that are interfering with our genetic make-up? How much damage to our DNA can the human body take before we can no longer reverse what we have been doing to ourselves? Perhaps all the illness in our world is a sign that we are on the wrong track. Americans spend more money on pharmaceutical drugs than any country in the world, yet we are the sickest country of all.

More and more of our children are obese, newlyweds are relying on fertility drugs to have children, and most adults are suffering from some sort of hormonal imbalance causing menstrual problems, sleep disturbances, adrenal failure, and depression as well as a host of other health issues.

In order to change our lives and to change our world, we all must start taking steps toward our health, one body at a time. We must learn to love again, starting with ourselves and extending to the entire planet. To love again means to stop consciously destroying and to start rebuilding what we have lost.

The time to rebuild is now. I invite you now to start your own journey, one step at a time. This is *your* life. *You* decide which path to follow.

If we want this world to be a better place, the time is now. One mouthful at a time.

Tracking Your Progress

CALIPER BODY FAT INTERPRETATION CHART

To use this chart, add up your three caliper readings and divide by three (This gives you your average glycogen reading in mm). Then find the mm number that is closest to your result. The number in the box will be your body fat percentage:

MALES

(mm)	5 6	7 8	9 10	11 12	13 14	15 16	17 18	19 20	21 22	23 24	25 26	27 28	29 30	31 32	33 34	35 36
<20	6.2	8.5	10.5	12.5	14.3	16.0	17.5	18.9	20.2	21.3	22.3	23.1	23.8	24.3	24.9	25.4
21-25	7.3	9.5	11.6	13.6	15.4	17.0	18.6	20.0	21.2	22.3	23.3	24.2	24.9	25.4	25.8	26.3
26-30	8.4	10.6	12.7	14.6	16.4	18.1	19.6	21.0	22.3	23.4	24.4	25.2	25.9	26.5	26.9	27.4
31-35	9.4	11.7	13.7	15.7	17.5	19.2	20.7	22.1	23.4	24.5	25.5	26.3	27.0	27.5	28.0	28.5
36-40	10.5	12.7	14.8	16.8	18.6	20.2	21.8	23.2	24.4	25.6	26.5	27.4	28.1	28.6	29.0	29.7
41-45	11.5	13.8	15.9	17.8	19.6	21.3	22.8	24.7	25.5	26.6	27.6	28.4	29.1	29.7	30.1	30.6
46-50	12.6	14.8	16.9	18.9	20.7	22.4	23.9	25.3	26.6	27.7	28.7	29.5	30.2	30.7	31.3	31.9
51-55	13.7	15.9	18.0	20.0	21.8	23.4	25.0	26.4	27.6	28.7	29.7	30.6	31.2	31.8	32.2	32.7
>56	14.7	17.0	19.1	21.0	22.8	24.5	26.0	27.4	28.7	29.9	30.8	31.6	32.3	32.9	33.3	34.0

AGE

FEMALES

(mm)	5 6	7 8	9 10	11 12	13 14	15 16	17 18	19 20	21 22	23 24	25 26	27 28	29 30	31 32	33 34	35 36
<20	15.7	17.7	19.7	21.5	23.2	24.8	26.3	27.7	29.0	30.2	31.3	32.3	33.1	33.9	34.6	35.3
21-25	16.3	18.4	20.3	22.1	23.8	25.5	27.0	28.4	29.6	30.8	31.9	32.9	33.8	34.5	35.2	35.8
26-30	16.9	19.0	20.9	22.7	24.5	26.1	27.6	29.0	30.3	31.5	32.5	33.5	34.4	35.2	35.8	36.5
31-35	17.6	19.6	21.5	23.4	25.1	26.7	28.2	29.6	30.9	32.1	33.2	34.1	35.0	35.8	36.4	37.0
36-40	18.2	20.2	22.2	24.0	25.7	27.3	28.8	30.2	31.5	32.7	33.8	34.8	35.6	36.4	37.0	37.6
41-45	18.8	20.8	22.8	24.6	26.3	27.9	29.4	30.8	32.1	33.3	34.4	35.4	36.3	37.0	37.7	38.4
46-50	19.4	21.5	23.4	25.2	26.9	28.6	30.1	31.5	32.8	34.0	35.0	36.0	36.9	37.6	38.3	39.0
51-55	20.0	22.1	24.0	25.9	27.6	29.2	30.7	32.1	33.4	34.6	35.6	36.6	37.5	38.3	38.9	39.6
>56	20.7	22.7	24.6	26.5	28.2	29.8	31.3	32.7	34.0	35.2	36.3	37.2	38.1	38.9	39.5	40.2

AGE

If your mm reading is higher than 36mm, divide your number by two and use the graph above.

The percent body fat will then be multiplied by two to determine your body fat percentage.

Example: If glycogen average was 40 mm for a 37-year-old female, divide 40 by two, which gives you 20 mm. Find the 20 mm mark at top of chart and 36-40 age on side of chart. These numbers intersect at 30.2% body fat. Then multiply that by two, which makes your current body fat at 60.4.

METABOLIC RATE FOR DAILY CALORIC REQUIREMENTS

Once you have determined your body fat percentage use this equation to find your actual fat pounds:

FAT WEIGHT = TOTAL POUNDS X % BODY FAT

Your fat free mass can then determined by using this equation:

FAT-FREE MASS = TOTAL POUNDS – FAT WEIGHT

Your fat-free mass is everything that is not fat in your body. This includes bone, organs, tissues, and lean muscle mass.

When determining your total calories consumption, we only want to use your fat-free mass in the next equation (We don't want to feed the fat!).

The graph below has already been adjusted to insure that you lose body fat, yet not so low that you would lose your lean body mass:

TOTAL CALORIES YOU NEED TO EAT EACH DAY:

	MALE	FEMALE
Sedentary	16 calories x fat free mass	15 calories x fat free mass
Light exercise	17 calories x fat free mass	16 calories x fat free mass
Moderate	18 calories x fat free mass	17 calories x fat free mass

To determine your goal weight, use this calculation:

GOAL WEIGHT = <u>LEAN BODY WEIGHT</u>
1.00 - % FAT DESIRED

If you are a 165-pound woman with a lean body weight of 100 pounds, wanting to be 20% body fat, your calculation would look like this:

$$\frac{100 \text{ pounds}}{1.00 - .20} = \frac{100 \text{ pounds}}{.80} = 125 \text{ pounds}$$

For those who would rather not do these calculations, you may use these basic calorie calculations:

WOMEN
- 80 - 100 lbs of lean muscle mass (LMM)
- Sedentary: 1120 – 1400 calories/day
- Active: 1440 – 1800 calories/day

MEN
- 100 -125 lbs of lean muscle mass (LMM)
- Sedentary: 1600 -2000 calories/day
- Active: 2100 – 2625 calories/day

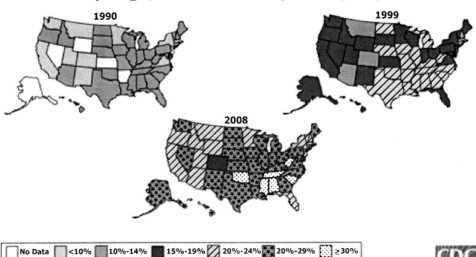

Obesity Trends* Among U.S. Adults
BRFSS, 1990, 1999, 2008
(*BMI ≥30, or about 30 lbs. overweight for 5'4" person)

| No Data | <10% | 10%-14% | 15%-19% | 20%-24% | 20%-29% | ≥30% |

Source: CDC Behavioral Risk Factor Surveillance System.

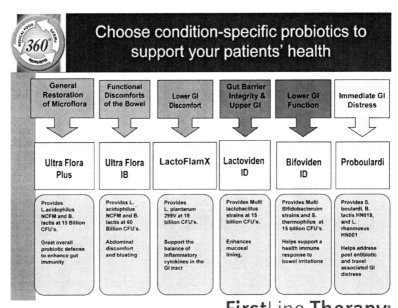

Choose condition-specific probiotics to support your patients' health

General Restoration of Microflora	Functional Discomforts of the Bowel	Lower GI Discomfort	Gut Barrier Integrity & Upper GI	Lower GI Function	Immediate GI Distress
Ultra Flora Plus	Ultra Flora IB	LactoFlamX	Lactoviden ID	Bifoviden ID	Proboulardi
Provides L.acidophilus NCFM and B. lactis at 15 Billion CFU's. Great overall probiotic defense to enhance gut immunity	Provides L. acidophilus NCFM and B. lactis at 60 Billion CFU's. Abdominal discomfort and bloating	Provides L. plantarum 299V at 18 billion CFU's. Support the balance of inflammatory cytokines in the GI tract	Provides Multi lactobacillus strains at 15 billion CFU's. Enhances mucosal lining,	Provides Multi Bifidobacteruim strains and S. thermophilus at 15 billion CFU's. Helps support a health immune response to bowel irritations	Provides S. boulardi, B. lactis HN019, and L. rhamnosus HN001 Helps address post antibiotic and travel associated GI distress

FirstLine Therapy®

EPA & DHA Supplementation

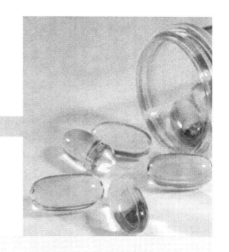

6:1 EPA:DHA Ratio Formulas

General EFA Supplementation

Anti Inflammatory

Metabolic Syndrome

Type 2 Diabetes

3:2 EPA:DHA Ratio Formulas

Combination Support

1:1 EPA:DHA Ratio Formulas

Cognitive Support

Prenancy and Nursing

Memory and Focus

Ratio of EPA to DHA	Serving Size	EPA	DHA
6:1 Ratio	1 softgel	500 mg	25-100 mg
3:2 Ratio	1 softgel	300 - 430 mg	200-290 mg
Concentrated Liquid (~3:2 Ratio)	1/4 tsp. (1.25ml)	350 mg	230 mg
1:1 Ratio Liquid	1/2 tsp. (2.5 ml)	300 mg	300 mg
Cod Liver Oil	1 tsp. (5 ml)	330 mg	460 mg

FirstLine Therapy is a registered trademark of Metagenics, Inc. © 2007

FirstLine Therapy°

TESTIMONIALS

Jeanette A.   Age 41
             Housewife and full-time student
             (Before I became a housewife I was a retail manager)

Before joining Angie's World my life was nearly paralyzed by my listless, fatigued and overweight body. In my late 30's I became a mother of two boys, a full-time student and a caregiver for my elderly mother. By the time I reached 40, I was consumed with stress and I found myself eating unbalanced meals on a regular basis. In an effort to regain my life, I tried every diet on the market only to face hunger and fuel my addiction to food. However, the worst crimes that I committed against my health were avoiding time for myself and facing my health issues with a defeatist attitude. I became married to baked goods, bleached flour and sugar rather than life.

My husband never understood how I was gaining weight because we ate daily as a family together, and we ate incredibly healthy meals. What he didn't see was my addiction to overeating baked goods and my late-night binges.

At the beginning of 2009 at the age of 40 I turned to Angie's World to help me regain a sustainable life of balanced eating and exercise. After a series of tests, I was faced with scientific proof that years of late-night eating, skipping meals, stress and a lack of exercise was affecting more than just my physical appearance. My health was in danger and as a mother and role model, my family's health was in danger. I found kind, caring and highly intelligent people at Angie's World who genuinely cared about my success and were pained by my situation. They constructed a new way of life for me: a balanced eating plan, a vitamin regimen, exercise, relaxation and necessary sleep. I never called the program at Angie's World a diet because the word diet conjured up fear, deprivation and failure. We focused on my fat and muscle percentages rather than the number on the scale and the eating plan was easy to follow and offered enough nutrition to avoid hunger.

Weight training was a new experience for me, especially free weights, and I was intimidated by the weight training area in the gym. We set up a weight training program that made me face my inhibition toward the free weight section and conquer my fears.

I simply followed the program, met my trainer and stuck to clean eating. Nobody is perfect and let's face it, a girl cannot live without chocolate. I will admit that I splurged a couple of times. I even accidentally ran into a pan of my homemade baklava once or twice. But as my body got stronger and leaner, I started bouncing back from occasional splurges faster. I realized that I could maintain my weight and fitness level if I just jumped back into the program. I have reached a sustainable lifestyle. I have lost 30 pounds and lowered my body fat by 9%. I am still on the program and I will continue until I have reached my desired weight and body composition. The most surprising reward from my experience with Angie's World is that I beat my addiction to food. And the most fulfilling reward is the healthy eating habits adopted by my family. Now at the dinner table we discuss how strong we are from eating healthy food and my boys don't only ask to see daddy's muscles, but mommy's muscles usually receive a *Wow!*

Tim H.   Age 72
                      Business owner
Since starting with Angie's World last year on my quest to shape up through diet and training, I have lost 20 pounds and have gained muscle and bone mass, which lead to a better outlook on life for myself and family. The nutritional diet has meant a smaller waist size (34 inches from 39 inches), and neck size (from 17 inches to 16 inches). My suit size changed from 42 short to 40 short. Of course, this has meant a lot of new clothes, but the compliments have made it all worthwhile. I have been going to the gym for the last 25 years and have been doing the wrong exercises the wrong way (according

to Angie), and growing fat. This has been corrected. On my initial interview with Angie, I told her of my double hernia operations and the pain I was still having and through her help and the right stretching exercises, the pain is gone.

Judy A.   Age 47
              Professional photographer
I am grateful for the lifestyle changes I have made with the guidance of my trainer. I have learned to make time to take care of myself. The action I take every day for myself has allowed me the confidence to pursue my dreams. We all know that exercise and eating right is what we have to do, but actually doing it can be a challenge. Coming up with excuses seems easier, but changing my mindset and thought pattern to doing it because it makes me feel good has improved every aspect of my life. I spent a lot of time coming up with excuses and, in hind-sight, that was actually more difficult.

Angie's notes: This next letter was written after she had experienced years of doctor's misdiagnosed treatments. They even suggested it was in her head. They removed her gall bladder and wanted to take her ovaries, but she said no. She is only 21 years old and has been dealing with chronic pain for over three years. We were able to determine that she had parasites, mostly from when she traveled to San Salvador. She gained over one hundred pounds in less than a year and couldn't keep any food down.

Ally A.   Age 21
              Student – Senior in college
Okay. Day 33 of the *health warrior project*. I owned oatmeal today. That is very exciting, seeing that I have been wretching or throwing up my food for months now. Blimpie lives on. I know now that that will soon subside. The buggies will die; I will rebuild my immune system and once again be myself. After all, my body only has three

more parasites to annihilate. Woo Hoo! It isn't always easy to be optimistic after having been sick for so long, but I really feel that I am doing what my body needs now. We certainly don't always see eye to eye. For example, I want to run errands, but my body has other plans like sleeping, watching another ridiculously awful but oddly entertaining *Charmed* marathon, or worshipping the porcelain god. I am making progress with the parasite protocol and organic living. IN fact I can't imagine where I WOULD BE WITHOUT THE TWO. So far this entire experience has taught me how to listen to my body and give it what it needs. Sometimes my body needs rest, sometimes it needs yoga, and when my body needs food it needs whole organic foods full of yummy nutrients. Every time I listen to my body now, I feel like I am rewarded with a feeling of contentment and an image of what my body will be able to do when I have helped it get healthy once again. I picture a slender, muscular body able to run, jump, laugh and do whatever I ask of it. OOOO, I am so excited!

Pam B.   Age 47
                        Vice President
November 2004
Going in for partial hysterectomy. I'm not going to gain weight. Everybody tells me that I will be gaining weight. I'm already close to 200 pounds and I can't do this anymore. I feel like I'm pregnant all over again. I have to get control of my life.

January 2005
Weighed in at 194. I need to lose about 50 pounds. I started working out with Angie three days a week and doing cardio in the evening with my friend Paula.

Mid 2005
Starting to see huge results, just need to keep this up. I learned these last few months that it isn't about willpower but about my attitude.

How bad do I want this? How bad do I want to change how I feel about myself? How bad do I want to be healthy? This is going to be about changing my habits forever, not just until I lose the weight. This change will be for the rest of my life.

Late 2005
A few girls in the office started Weight Watchers. They are excited but I truly don't think that a point system is going to make you healthy. Yes, it will help you lose weight but they are still eating everything and anything. I guess if at the end of the day you still have 100 points, you can eat anything you want, even cake and ice cream. It's all about the points!

2006
The girls are losing weight on Weight Watchers. Everybody has mentioned how good they look but I'm not sure why nobody says anything to me. At this time I've lost almost 50 pounds and no comments from anyone. I've said to myself that I need to understand that I'm not doing this for them. I'm doing this for me and it doesn't matter how many people say anything. I need to concentrate on me.

2007
Still have maintained my weight loss. I've learned so much about nutrition and exercise from Angie's World! Whatever Angie says, I *do*. I know that if I keep in the back of my mind that this is the way to lose weight I can *keep* it off. Exercise and nutrition are the keys. Girls at the office are off Weight Watchers for the last few months. I've already noticed one of them gaining her weight back, eating everything that she wants to and still not understanding what she needs to do.

2008
Still maintaining my weight loss and feeling pretty good. I've come to a plateau for the last several months but it's okay. I know that I'm eating good and exercising and maintaining my weight loss.

Still want to lose 10 more pounds but for some reason just can't get there. One of the girls at the office is now looking into gastric by-pass. She is taking a series of classes and after she completes those she is scheduled for surgery later this year. She has gained back the 70 pounds that she lost with Weight Watchers and has gained an additional 30 pounds. Everybody in the office is so proud of her because she will be skinny (after the gastric bypass) and that's what she deserves. I just don't get it! She knows that she can lose the weight with proper eating and exercise! The surgery still doesn't teach a person to eat healthy. It just means that she can still have a greasy taco but only eat half of it.

February 2009
Still maintaining my weight loss, a bit of a struggle these days be-cause I had the rest of my female organs removed which brought me into instant menopause. The doctor put me on Premarin right after the surgery, and he said that it is something that I will need to get me through this phase of my life.

March 2009
Asked my doctor if I need to stay on Premarin. I don't want to take it anymore. I don't have side effects, but I just don't like taking medication. He said that I could try but I might be very irritable and have hot flashes. I told him that I was going to try it and with Angie's help I weaned myself off the medication.

July 2009
Still struggling with my hormones but I just need to figure out that I need to increase my workouts and eat really clean to get over this change in my body. Five months later I'm still not taking any medi-cation for my hormones and I've had huge success with a natural product from Metagenics that has helped me get through this. After five years of maintaining my weight loss I know what I need to do and it's really so easy! It's a change in your attitude, caring about yourself, and changing your habits now and forever.

Jerry G.   Age 70

Retired from University of California, Riverside
I am happy to report that my family has always been sensitive to eating and exercising correctly but still I was heavier than I wanted to be, and could not reduce. Finally, I made the decision to meet with Angie to determine what could be adjusted in order to accomplish my goal. After going through her tests she told me that I could easily lose 20 pounds using her exercise program and following her diet. What really sold me was that her diet contained good quality food and did not include special diet products often found with the many fat-loss programs. Indeed, I was skeptical but very interested and signed up for 12 weeks. At the rate of about one and one half pounds per week, I lost those 20 pounds by the end of three months. I continue to follow the diet, eating lots of fresh, and often organic, vegetables, cutting back on bad carbs, and increasing my protein. Three months have gone by since ending my program with Angie and her wonderful assistant, Wilma, and I am still at my new weight. Actually I would like to lose five more pounds and know how to do it, but with Angie, Wilma my trainer, and the entire Angie's World Staff looking over my shoulder, that goal would be more reachable, I am sure.
The downside of all this is having to buy new summer pants and storing those that are now too big. The plus side is my ability to wear those good quality slacks that have been hanging in the closet for a few years waiting for that magic time when they would fit again. They are magicians!

Estelle S.   Age 81

Model - retired
After entering Angie's World two years ago as a tired, worn-out eighty-year-old and taking part in her exercise, vitamin and nutrition programs, I am now a sixty-year-old woman (working on fifty), who is strong and healthy. Angie is the fountain of youth.
P.S. I dumped my 80-year-old husband and have a 40-year-old boyfriend.

126

But seriously, I never realized how important eating the right foods, in the right combinations is for your health. I never was a bad eater, but I never realized how little protein I was eating. Since I started this program, I have more energy, I am sick a whole lot less, and my posture has improved tremendously. I used to think it was just the way you are supposed to feel and look when you get older but now I know it has more to do with what I eat and whether or not I am exercising.

Rosemary N.   Age 51
                       Teacher

As I reflect on the journey that started for me two-and-a-half years ago, I can't help but recall a recurring theme: perseverance. When I began I was 49 years old with an eight-year-old daughter who needed a mom who could keep up with her and enjoy life with her as an active parent. I knew that my health was about to become severely compromised with diabetes and heart disease if I didn't get serious about taking good care of myself. I was a professional short-term dieter who always garnered great results. The problem was that the results were short-term as well. I came to Angie with great hope, excitement, and a determined attitude. I knew the journey I was gearing up for would be long, and at time, probably painful. The journey has not let my expectations down. Scattered among the successes were plateaus that were frustrating and disheartening. Many times I questioned myself and felt like giving up. It was at those times that physical or emotional change was about to occur and I just needed to keep my head down and persevere. Angie would always know exactly what to say and recommend to put me back on tract, and within a few weeks I would be showing positive results once again. This journey isn't over; it never will be. What I started two-and-a-half years ago was the beginning of my new life. I am stronger, healthier, and more alive than I have ever been. I have accomplished my goal of being an active parent. During the journey my daughter and I earned a first-degree black belt in Taekwondo together; I have successfully hiked some grueling mountain peaks; and I am about to run my first 5K race. Perseverance has been the theme, as it will be for the remainder of my life. I can do anything if I persevere!

Mady H.   Age 61
                     Accountant

I've considered myself fit and have been eating healthy for the past 15 years or so. My parents both had colon cancer so I knew of the dangers of too much fat and grease. In 2007 I discovered I had breast cancer and had a lumpectomy along with chemotherapy and radiation treatment. Of course, now I really had to take care of myself. I wanted to be healthy, not have a recurrence of cancer, and live a long life.

A few months ago, my energy level was very low and I didn't feel like exercising as much as I had, being tired after working all day. I would walk but not much else. I was constantly craving sweets and indulging in cookies only here or there but enough that when I ate one, I wanted another. I felt in a rut and what else could I do? Knowing Angie as a personal friend and having some guidance through the years on nutrition, I decided to go ahead and have a full nutrition analysis with her and get myself back on course to living healthy and feeling better all around.

It has been only four weeks of following the First Line Therapy Program she set me on and I am feeling great. I wasn't in it for the weight loss especially but I did lose five pounds and lost inches all over without any feelings of hunger. After the first three days my energy level was up and I had no sweet cravings! I started exercising 30-45 minutes daily plus my 40-minute daily walk. I never felt deprived of food and sometimes felt I was eating too much because of the full feeling. I found out how little protein I was eating for my body and along with the combination of fruits, vegetables and good grains and legumes, I have energy to spare.

The first week was actually fun to see the combinations I could put together to get all the food groups in my day. My husband called me the mad scientist in the kitchen nightly preparing for the next day. I wanted to be sure of the right amounts and variety to eat and I figured that Angie would be checking up on me in four weeks, so I didn't want to *not* show progress. Most of all I didn't want let myself down and needed to prove that I could change myself even though I always thought I was a healthy eater. I look forward in the next four weeks to meeting my goals and, of course, looking and feeling better each day. At 60 years old, it is never too late to improve physically and do the activities I've always loved. I'll be water-skiing next weekend!

Janis B.   Age 66
                      Childcare Provider

I lost two of my younger brothers and my mother in a short 17 months several years ago. Both brothers died at the age of 48 years old. The first brother had had bypass surgery but he didn't change his eating habits or lifestyle and died of a heart attack a year later. The other brother died 17 months later. After spending a week in Hawaii with the rest of my family I was having a hard time walking, my face would get red and I would get short of breath. I weighed around 230 pounds. My older brother said he was worried about me and if I didn't do something about my weight I would be the next to die. It really opened my eyes.

I have been going to Angie's World for almost three years. After my first month with her I only lost a small amount of weight. I knew Angie meant business because she really got on my case. WOW! Did she open my eyes! She had me start writing down everything I ate and sending it to her weekly, but after a few weeks of not doing too well, she had me send my menus to her daily because I was having a hard time keeping myself honest and being accountable.

At times I didn't want to face Angie, but I knew if I was going to get healthy, I had to listen to her and do what she said. She holds me accountable for every bit I put in my mouth. I have tried every diet in the book from diet pills to shots and every ad you see on TV. I have never in my life stuck with a plan as long as I have with Angie. I know it's for life and not a short-term diet like I've done in the past. Now I read every label before I buy anything. This time I really think it's about trying to keep myself healthy. It's not a diet. It's a new and healthy way of life. I really feel I have accomplished so much in the last three years.

I have wanted to give up so many times but Angie always says the right thing to keep me going and I thank her for that! She has taught me so much about food and how important it is to read labels. Also how important exercise is to keep me healthy.

Paula W.   Age 45
             Financial Branch Manager

It's been three-and-a-half years of Angie in my life and still going. I have learned to change my eating lifestyle and how I look at food. Let me tell you the journey has not been easy. There have been days, many days, I didn't want to get out of bed to go and train. Of course when I get there Angie is always in such an upbeat and happy mood she can't wait to put a hurtin' on my body. And you know it's bad when I'm working out and she is pushing me so hard my eyelids start to sweat! You try and get some sympathy but it doesn't work. She just pushes you on to the next set of exercises and many times I close my eyes and then take a peek through one eye hoping and wishing she would be gone but she is still there pushing me and guiding me to make the right choices. I am 80 pounds lighter and have kept the weight off for a year and a half and I am feeling great. It's a lifetime choice. I have chosen to fuel my body with better choices of food and add daily exercise. Thank you, Angie, for helping me through my weight loss journey. I will always be grateful.

Al C.   Age 42
UC Riverside Staff

I've learned a lot working out with Angie and I really get a lot better use out of the gym. But even better I am eating a whole lot healthier than I used to because of Angie's nutritional counseling. I feel that her "diet" is just good common sense that I can use for the rest of my life. I certainly feel a lot better.

Mitchell M.   Age 26
Sales Representative

After I had knee surgery, I ballooned up to 230 pounds with about 30% body fat and I looked a mess. But thanks to you and all the advice on nutrition and workouts, my body has gone through dramatic changes. I now weigh 174 pounds and my body fat is at 8.8%.

Colleen B.   Age 56
Director of Human Resources

My story is simple. I worked with Angie's World, not only to find an exercise regimen but to learn more about eating right. I've lost weight, and held that loss for over two years now. While I am not at my ideal weight, I know I can and *will* move forward. Exercise, focus, and good nutrition are what it is all about. Simple, true, and productive. It helps to have a coach and someone who helps with accountability.

Missi R.   Age 65
Nurse -retired

In a recent article on aging, the physician writing their article stated a personal trainer is good because she is upbeat, encouraging and makes sure you are exercising properly and safely. That's why I continue going to Angie. She's upbeat, encouraging and knowledgeable about nutrition as well as exercise and she is definitely FUN!! Under her training, I have maintained my weight and continued to build lean muscle mass. For someone 65, that is really a plus!! For women over 50, weight lifting is among the best things we can do to not only maintain lean muscle but to maintain our total musculo-skeletal health. Bone health is of utmost importance in this age group and weight lifting helps us gain bone, muscle and balance, all of which help in the prevention of falls. It is a win-win situation.

A bi-weekly session with my trainer is what keeps me on track with both my nutrition and fitness. Without the continual nutrition reminders and how it works along with my exercise to keep me toned, I would find it very difficult to maintain my weight. It is the regularity of the sessions with my trainer that has made a real difference in my progress. I need the mental boost and the educational input to keep me interested in reaching my fitness goals.

Angela D.   Age 55
            Retired executive from NASA Ames Research
            Center in Silicon Valley
            Executive Coach

My journey into Angie's World started approximately 1 year ago. I had moved to the Riverside area and was determined to find a trainer to help me get back to a healthy exercise schedule to tone up and increase my stamina. A friend had recommended Angie. I've worked with various trainers on the East Coast and West coach and without a doubt, Angie is the best I've trained with over the past 15 years. The reason is the combination of training and nutrition. This holistic approach has helped me achieve steady progress and results in achieving my goals. The training is focused, professional, timely and motivating, plus it's fun. Angie has this unique quality of working you to your fullest potential (always just one more rep or adding five more pounds), while making it fun (sharing stories and laughing a lot). And the nutrition counseling and biomeridian assessment tool have been instrumental in identifying challenges (heavy metal) and tracking healthy qualities (muscle mass, hydration). Even though I've recently moved out of state, I still train with Angie when I'm in Riverside, have my biomeridian, and replenish my supplements. Angie is a knowledgeable, caring and perseverant nutritionist who is constantly increasing her certifications and professional competencies. I am grateful for her guidance, instruction, and encouragement.

Diana R.   Age 68
                     Medical office manager -retired
Angie is amazing! I always feel better once I've done a session with her. It's her positive attitude and energy towards life that makes her a joy to be around. She inspires you to improve in ALL aspects of life. Her workout program is an important part of my life.

Ernie S.   Age 51
                     CEO
I came to Angie's World at 226 pounds, drinking tons of coffee and quickly aging my body and my mind. In 4 short months with their help and direction I have lost 30 pounds, become mentally sharper, and have added years to my life. Their plan is based on a camaraderie of working together of building my knowledge on nutrition and exercise, guiding me on the choices that a hectic life provides, and teaching me to navigate the healthiest possibilities. I am eternally grateful to Angie and her team for giving me the gift of health!

Peggy K   Age 28
                     Graduate Student
I'd like to commend you for the work that you are doing. As a graduate student studying health psychology, I study the long-term effects of health-related behaviors on health, well-being, and longev-

ity. Living a healthy lifestyle - exercise, diet, managing stress, good social relationships, etcetera are essential, not only for short term benefit, but throughout your life. It's exciting to see that you are helping people put these elements into practice.

I'd also like to thank you for your influence on my own life. As a long-distance runner, being active has not been a problem for me, but I was not a healthy runner. I did not realize how important nutrition, sleep, and stress management are to my health and performance. I recently ran the Carlsbad Marathon (26.2 miles). Despite my training, I neglected the nutritional component, which led to a debilitating injury that completely derailed my training, making me wonder if I'd even be able to complete the race. Through your help, I was able to not only gain back the muscle mass that I had lost through my own poor diet choices and build strength for the race, but also ran an excellent race, finishing in just over 3 hours as the second place woman!

The marathon experience was a good start. I have much to learn, more changes to make. But I am confident in what I am learning from you, and look forward to what the future holds.

Thank you, from the bottom of my heart.

Glenda G.   Age 54
                      Business owner
I have Rheumatoid Arthritis, had "Total Knee Replacement" on my right knee, and later had surgery for tendon repair. When you have a disease that limits a lot of what you can and can't do, it really makes it difficult to decide to do anything. Swimming was my only friendly exercise. My doctors have been telling me for years that I needed to exercise regularly and I kept coming up with excuses about how much it hurt. Would you believe it, they were right. Angie's World set me up with three virtual workouts: Upper Body, Lower Body and one for Shoulders and Back. I feel great and I'm still losing weight and building muscle I weigh less now than I did when I got married

23 years ago, and according to Angie's wonder machine my age is 27. So, I not only weigh less I'm younger.......I'm in so much better shape thanks to Angie's World and my husband who is my coach. I'm even doing cycling classes with him!

Karen L.   Age 32
                 Hairdresser

Thank you for educating me on health and fitness. I have always been an active person and what I thought was fairly healthy, until you sat me down and really educated me on my diet and weight training. You have really instilled some new values in me about how to take care of myself through eating right and exercise. Now I am able to get the most out of my workouts and definitely see quicker results. I thank you for really getting me to respect my body and what I can make it look like! My confidence is way up, and I love the way I look!!

Marshall S.   Age 73
                    Insurance Agent

Over the years I have had a number of trainers and none were very effective. Under your tutelage I made great strides and after a stem cell transplant you brought me back where I was before and maybe a little beyond that! You are the best!!!

Sarah W.   Age 26
                 Secretary

I was worried how I would look on my wedding day. I had started to get lazy and was spending too much time in the drive-thru. With only two months until the wedding I was starting to panic; then I found Angie's World. Angie was kind and caring and helped me to pinpoint all my diet and exercise mistakes. She helped me to manage my diet adding more protein to my diet as well as vitamins my body had been lacking. I have been doing weight training with Angie's World twice weekly and have watched my body change into a leaner more sculpted body. Everyone is noticing as I have melted from a size thirteen to a four. The best part is how great I feel; I have so much more energy and stamina. My confidence has gone through the roof! I want to thank Angie's World again for all of their support and guidance. I have had to return my wedding dress twice to a smaller size and I will be proud to walk down the aisle.

Kia G.   Age 30
                Business professional & mother

My friend introduced me to Angie's World on my 30th birthday as a present. She knew I wanted to get back in shape after my second child turned two. I was always in good shape and had exercised regularly but could not lose the "baby fat." My old exercise regimen included aerobics 3-4 times a week and eating a decent vegetarian diet. What I learned from Angie's World was that I needed a cleaner diet (i.e. less carbs and sugar and more protein). They combined that with weight training - something I had NEVER done before. I learned a lot about what types and amount of exercise yields the best results and what a large role food has in achieving these results. With their help, within 5 months I had been "transformed" and entered my first competition where I placed 4th!!! I lost 22 pounds and gained more muscle than I have ever had. I feel and look wonderful! Angie's World is truly amazing. I couldn't have done it without them.

Ed B.   Age 33
                Businessman

I can tell you honestly getting started with my transformation was not an easy task. Being a workaholic this took a total adjustment of lifestyle. Making time for the gym, and it may sound funny, but making time to actually eat!! At first I was working out 2 - 3 times a week for 30 minutes and not seeing any results. Not looking to become an Arnold Schwarzenegger type, I just wanted to shed some weight, gain muscle definition, and increase my strength and endurance. Angie's World educated me on the importance of nutrition. I was eating all of the wrong foods with little or no protein. Once I started eating clean foods along with the proper supplements I noticed results in only a few days. I could actually see muscles forming, clothes began to fit looser and looser. Let me tell you that there is not a more gratifying feeling than to have to go shopping for new clothes because your old clothes are too big. Showing off a six-pack is pretty awesome too!

Maria I.   Age 55
                     Medical Interpreter
My life has changed and I have become an inspiration to my friends who believed because we are over 50 we are doomed to look our age as well as feel old. My personal goal has set a precedent; the people around me can see losing weight and staying healthy can be a reality and not just a dream.

Carrie M.   Age 39
                     Pharmaceutical Rep
When I needed to get in shape for my wedding, Angie's World was the answer. Their enthusiasm for fitness and constant encouragement helped me stay focused and determined. Angie's World personalized my fitness goals and took an active role in making sure I achieved them. They were a constant reminder that my hard work and persistence would indeed pay off. Whenever I needed a boost, they had something new for me. Whether it was a new exercise, recipe or diet tip, Angie's excitement and knowledge of fitness kept me motivated. I was able to achieve great results, quickly, by following their recommendations and advice. I am truly thankful for the guidance and vision. They can-and will-help you reach your fitness goals.

Joyce C.   Age 36
           Computer Specialist
A coworker (an acquaintance for about 15 years) told me that working with Angie's World has totally changed me. Apparently I seem a lot happier, less tired and more talkative and social. I don't talk in such a quiet voice and when I talk now, it's not just about computer stuff that no one else understands. Hehe. That's good! But, I'm still a computer geek. LOL

Sandy S.   Age 46
           Financial Planner
I feel very fortunate that I have never really had a weight problem but I really wanted to be toned. When I started with Angie's World last year, my main goals were to get definition in my arms and to tone my stomach. I am now reaching my goals, having fun doing it and loving the results. Angie is a great motivator and supporter.

Jonathan B.   Age 37
           Nephrologist
Angie's World has helped me understand the importance of being consistent with exercise and nutrition. I have better knowledge of clean eating and exercise. They have helped me establish reasonable goals for a lifetime of health. I am far from where I want to be but with Angie's World, I am on the right path.

Carole G.   Age 69
           Vice President
I've been working out with Angie's World for 10 months. I look & feel better & stronger than I did 10 years ago.

Endnotes

[1] Winter, Ruth M.S, 1999. *A Consumer's Dictionary of Food Additives: Fifth Addition,* Three Rivers Press, New York.

Print References

Appleton, Ph.D. Nancy, *146 Reasons Why Sugar is Ruining your Health,* www.nancyappleton.com. (author of Lick the Sugar Habit).

Blaylock, MD, Russel L, 1997, *Excitotoxins: The Taste that Kills,* Health Press, Santa Fe, NM.

FirstLineTherapy, 2006. *Therapeutic Lifestyle Program. For Better Health Now and for a Lifetime,* Rev. 06.06 Advanced Nutrition Publications, Inc.

Metagenics, 2006. *Simple & Easy Detoxification,* Advanced Nutrition Publications, Inc.

van den Heuvel, E., et al. 1999 *Oligofructose stimulates calcium absorption in adolescents.* American Journal of Clinical Nutrition 69(March):544-548. Available at http://www.ajcn.org/cgi/content/full/69/3/544

Winter, Ruth M.S, 2009. *A Consumer's Dictionary of Food Additives: Seventh Addition,* Three Rivers Press, New York.

Zafar, T.A., C.M. Weaver, et al. 2004. Nondigestible oligosaccharides increase calcium absorption and suppress bone resorption in ovariectomized rats. Journal of Nutrition 134 (February):399-402. Abstract available at http://jn.nutrition.org/cgi/content/abstract/134/2/399

Selected Electronic Media References

www.plucodes.com/docs/IFPS-plu_codes_users_guide.pdf
http://rheumatic.org/sugar.htm
www.truvia.com
www.benefits-of-honey.com
www.wikipedia.org
http://stress.about.com/c/ec/1.htm
http://www.clevelandclinic.org/health
http://www.bodyandmind.co.za/healthweb/The_Importance_of_
Streching.html
http://www.healthandyoga.com/html/yoga/Benefits.html
http://www.scorecard.org
http://www.chelationtherapyonline.com/technical/p8.htm
http://www.pureinsideout.com/fasting-for-detox.html
http://www.holidays.net/highholydays/yom.htm
http://www.epa.gov/superfund/programs/recycle/faqs/index.html#1
http://www.scorecard.org
http://oracvalues.com
www.brunswicklabs.com
www.drmercola.com
http://dsc.discovery.com/videos/news-honey-bee-killer-hunted.html

BODY BY ANGIE

Step onto the right path, create a positive force in your life,
and improve your health!

Sign up for our **free** online newsletter and stay informed
with our products, upcoming events, exercise and nutrition tips.

Visit **angiesworld.com** for more nutritional and fitness strategies.

Remember, it is a journey you are undertaking not a
destination, and I am here to help steer and guide you.

May health and happiness be yours!

- Angie

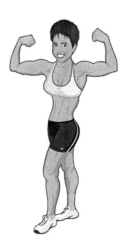

If I can do it, so can you!

Angie Lustrick, CN, CPT
Certified Nutritionist and ACSMCertified Personal Trainer

Angie Lustrick is a certified nutritionist and an ACSM certified personal trainer. She received her Bachelor's degree in Biology at the University of California, Riverside and her Master's degree in nutrition at American Health Science University. Angie is the President of Angie's World - a personal training and nutrition center located in Riverside. Angie is a professional public speaker and has made numerous appearances in print and live media. Recently, Angie filmed a miniseries for PBS-KVCR on Hispanic Lifestyles in which she gives nutritional and exercise advice. In the past, Angie has also been heard or seen on NPR radio, Spencer PowerHour, Personal TrainerTV.com, HealthyLife. net, SpikeTV and many more. She has produced two exercise videos and has developed a line of personal skin care products.

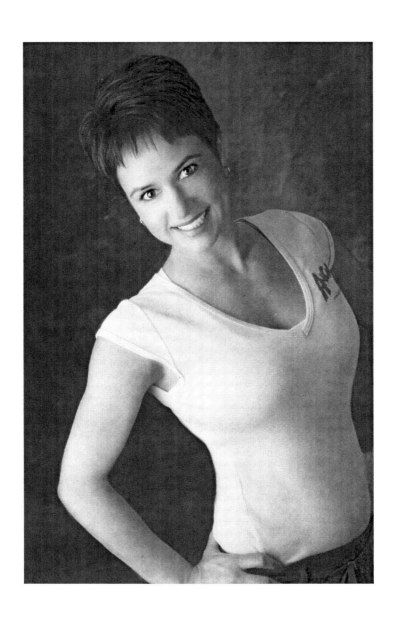

LaVergne, TN USA
18 June 2010
186618LV00004B/25/P